Home Is Where I Live

The future enters us in this way in order to be transformed itself in us, long before it happens.*
—Rainer Maria Rilke

Home Is Where I Live

Camilla Warrick

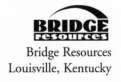

Bridge Resources
Louisville, Kentucky

Unless otherwise noted, Scripture quotations are from the New Revised Standard Version of the Bible, copyright © 1989 by the Division of Christian Education of the National Council of the Churches of Christ in the U.S.A. Used by permission.

Every effort has been made to trace copyrights on the materials included in this book. If any copyrighted material has nevertheless been included without permission and due acknowledgment, proper credit will be inserted in future printings after notice has been received.

Edited by Beth Basham

Book interior and cover design by Kim House

First edition

Published by Bridge Resources
Louisville, Kentucky

Web site address: http://www.bridgeresources.org

PRINTED IN THE UNITED STATES OF AMERICA

99 00 01 02 03 04 05 06 07 08 — 10 9 8 7 6 5 4 3 2 1

Warrick, Camilla, date.
    Home is where I live / Camilla Warrick. —1st ed.
        p.   cm.
    ISBN 1-57895-040-6
    1. Cancer—Patients—Religious life. 2. Warrick, Camilla, 1954—Diaries.
    3. Cancer—Patients—United States—Diaries. I. Title.
    BV4910.33.W37 2000
    362.1'96994'0092—dc21   99-037020

I dedicate this to those who seek
and those who help seekers find.

Contents

Preface

This is a selfish little book.

The selfish big book consists of many black-bound journals, squeezed into bookshelves in our home. The contents are raw, often angry, totally unedited, tied together with loopy arrows and margin notes intended for nobody but me—unless I decide otherwise. Can you hear that strident tone? Can you see me with hands on hips?

Indeed, the first page of every journal announces "Private" in large letters. Sometimes, too, "Keep Out."

I need to claim a lot of space to be selfish. But at $1.49 a volume, these journals I pick up at the grocery store are real estate's best bargain.

By *selfish* I don't mean "void of regard for others," the secondary meaning of the word. But I do mean, "chiefly regarding one's own self." Dare I say it? Become selfish and you will heal.

I could save you the time spent reading this little book by telling you that the only thing that matters is process—and not a single process. For me, it may be my odd ruminations with a pen. For another, it may be making music. For a third, carving wood. For many more, it is found in a mix of idioms and with a mash of creations.

For a few, I imagine, prayer alone is their most selfish act. Not other people's prayers, but a nonverbal, unclenched expression of vulnerability, exposed like a flame before God.

If you cannot take time for yourself, if you can't listen, if you have no regard for the peculiarities of your own energy, passion, and attachments, how can you expect to live? Where will you ever find someone who can love you more than you are willing to love yourself?

Dare I say more? Anything short of self-love involves addiction. And by that, I mean a willingness to be duped, to settle for substitutes, to avoid the heart's deepest craving.

But don't take my word for it. I would hardly expect that.

This little book came into being when I stopped taking other people at their word. Things were already stirred up in my life, so I felt a license to turn over assumptions and beliefs, to feel my own feelings and speak my own words. I can remember the dark November morning when I walked out to my car to go to work, looked up at the stars, and knew in an instant what I had to do.

I had to write down my understanding of healing, and I had to do it soon. I felt this with an urgency that makes sense to me, but is difficult to explain sensibly. And yet, the people most likely to be affected—my husband, children, boss, dearest friends—nodded and smiled and said okay.

I requested a four-month leave from my journalism job. Paul Knue, editor of *The Cincinnati Post*, gave me that and more. He supported the endeavor and suggested that I turn part of my searchings into a series for the paper. Whatever I did with the rest of it was my business.

When the words began to tumble, I distrusted them at first. I heard a new voice speaking. Was this my voice? After several weeks of surrender, writing without an outline, a beginning, middle, or end, I began to relax. This was medicine I needed, medicine only I could give myself.

Perhaps this form of selfishness can be discovered alone, pursued without guilt and enjoyed without the encouragement of family, coworkers, mentors, or friends. But I lacked the courage. I needed those people who would say, "This is precious. This is necessary. Do it."

Hence, I reflect on those people, who did that for me, with great gratitude. I can think of no more lasting gift to give other people than tiny shoves of trust or enthusiasm that make it possible for them to begin expressing a silent part of themselves.

My dream for this book is that it could do the same. But championing process isn't always enough. Nor is a cheer of trust and enthusiasm. Practical concerns can pose real difficulties.

I don't know what you need or what it will take to get you started, but I offer my help in this way:

— Seventy percent of my proceeds from this book will go into a fund to help you or someone you know live more fully.

— I will attach as few strings as possible to its use.

— Stipends will be for female or male, young or old, sick or well.

— I will look for other opportunities to beef up the fund and have a nonprofit board oversee it.

In the event that sales are stale, I will take the money and buy journals. Who knows, purchased in bulk they might be had for just ninety-nine cents. I will hand them out like slices of bread. I may toss in one of my favorite roller-ball pens, and I will inquire whether you have an adequate flashlight next to your bed.

All I know is that when the pain awakens, the words will follow. They will take you inward and outward, and they may take you away from words altogether. But you must know, now and always, this is precious. This is necessary. Do it.

Morning

I stand before a mirror and try to wink my right eye. Getting nowhere, I wink my left. No problem. Then I hold open my left eye, insisting that it not wink, and go back to work on my right. I turn my head to the left and try it again, isolating muscles.

Some days I try to raise my ring finger. I ask it to stand up, solo, while all the others are held down. It cannot.

"When I figure out how to do this, I'm going to have great ball control in soccer," I tell the boys.

"Right, Mom." They don't believe in this kind of magic.

Some days I set the microwave on two minutes and watch the digital seconds count down. They move precisely, of course. But slowly, it seems. I try not to fidget. I'm going to get there. I'm going to make it to zero. I haven't yet.

I can't remember ever not winking my left eye. I can't remember not whistling or rolling my tongue into a loud ring. I can't remember not blowing gum into bubbles.

But surely there was a time when I could not. Then came a day when impulses regrouped and I crossed from not doing to doing.

I am waiting for that day, courting it in a kingdom of words. I am searching for the questions that will make all my answers dazzle.

Elie Wiesel says, "The space between any two words is vaster than the distance between heaven and earth."[1]

But I have too many words and too little space. They gush out of me, gaining volume and momentum each day. I fill journal after journal. "Boil, little pot, boil." My streets are full of porridge. It rises like a river, and I have forgotten the spell to make it stop.

---

1. From *All Rivers Run to the Sea* by Elie Wiesel, p. 321. Copyright © 1995 by Alfred A. Knopf, Inc. Reprinted by permission of the publisher.

I was raised on the notion of a life span, stretching like a spear from base to tip. Yet I also was raised on those disembodied beginnings of fables, "Once upon a time." I coursed the living room to the singsong of A. A. Milne:

> I think I am an Elephant,
>
> Behind another Elephant
>
> Behind *another* Elephant who isn't really there.
>
> . . . So *round* about
>
> And *round* about
>
> And *round* about and *round* about
>
> And *round* about
>
> And *round* about I go.[2]

My belief in time's linear advance was eroded by cycles of the moon, by dreams that wouldn't go away, by the woman who handed me a banquet program on Saturday night, and I recognized it, as if from long ago. My name was on it.

"You will need to announce that Jane is sick," she said.

I nodded. I feel as if I've been here before. I know it.

Today a book arrived in the mail. It had a return address, the Institute of Noetic Sciences in Sausalito, California. I'm familiar with that place. I love the book inside. But I had not ordered it, and nothing indicated why it was sent. Yet two days ago this was the book, Rachel Remen's *Kitchen Table Wisdom*, that I gave to a friend to give to her friend. I had to swallow first. I don't part with treasures easily.

So I write: To make sense of it all. To speak my truth.

I return to the familiar and the linear, to the journals I keep. I remind myself, this isn't the beginning. It's just a moment in a circle of days.

---

2. From *Now We Are Six* by A. A. Milne (New York: Puffin Books, 1927), p. 10. Copyright renewed in 1955 by A. A. Milne.

Afternoon

August 19, 1996

"It's cancer." The words, spoken by a surgeon this morning, are still ringing in my ears. Maybe they always will. I don't blame anyone, except maybe, a little, myself.

But I'm not looking for scapegoats. Only angels. They are here: A good hug from Betsy; Paul trying hard to be tender; Hal here; boys gentle, though too distant.

Maybe this will help me set inconsequential things aside. I hope the process is full of poetry. I will let the words spill and tears tumble, if they must. Only if they must.

I don't want to exist out of this wound. I don't want to be defined by this disease.

I feel as if I've hardly even lived. Yet I have lived so long, so well. A life of comfort, ease, great groceries, pretty good wine. I am praying for fear to fall away. To sweat again from good, hard exertion. Ah, to sweat again.

A little peace is coming, flowing over me.

I still have to make decisions. Still have to make phone calls, set up appointments, tell friends and family, inviting them to fight this with me—open and patient.

I want to live for the boys, to mother them, cheer for them, watch them grow taller, listen to their wisdom deepen.

I want to lose my roughness, better understand everything, and grow a softer, bigger heart.

I want it all—the sweet music that rises into the night sky, reaching the stars; the cold water that cleanses; the books I have not read; the prayers that transform. Maybe some more good meals. No! Lots of good meals. I want to share everything and spend a little impulsively.

Two days later the tumor and the breast that concealed it were removed and sent to the lab. "Preoperative diagnosis: carcinoma of the left breast. Postoperative diagnosis: same. Labeled 'left breast' is a 17 x 16 x .5 cm. left breast having an overlying 19 x 6 cm. tan wrinkled skin ellipse and a 7 x 6 x 2.5 cm. attached axillary fat pad." And so forth.

I could imagine the pathologist picking over it with gloved hands and a small scalpel. She sipped a Diet Coke and dictated her findings into a tape recorder. "There is an approximately 5 cm. in greatest dimension firm, tan-gray, ill-defined area located adjacent to the biopsy cavity in the upper quadrant that grossly involves three quadrants. This firm area has multiple diffuse pinpoint foci that exude a creamy tan-yellow material."

Yuck.

"Infiltrating ductal carcinoma, histologic grade II. Extensive intraductal carcinoma of cribriform and comedo type." And so forth. "Metastatic carcinoma in nine of eleven axillary lymph nodes with extranodal extension. Left subpectoral lymph node: metastatic carcinoma consistent with breast primary in one of one lymph node."

I say, "Cancer has taken me on a journey." But *journey* has become flabby from overfeeding. Put "spiritual" in front of it, and it's like tapping one of those preprogrammed keys on a computer, merging five processes into one. A message blinks onto the screen: "Congratulations. You have just removed yourself from the confines of ordinary people and are now breathing air piped in from the Himalayas."

Ah, how important I am.

I search for another expression. "Cancer has served as a catalyst." But strictly speaking a *catalyst* is an agent that initiates action between two or more persons or forces and "itself remains unaffected by the action."

Unaffected? My cancer? I hope not.

So I return to the cliché: "Cancer has taken me on a journey." It has ignited my spirit. But I am not removed from ordinary people or breathing rarefied air. I am ordinary, and I am breathing, and this process is ordinary human entitlement.

I used to think this journey was activated by breast cancer—the fallout from a collision between outward circumstances and inward vulnerability. For women like me, who are between the ages of 35 and 50, breast cancer has the feel of a plague. Our second leading killer, breast cancer growing out of control claims more than 46,000 of us annually. As others have pointed out, this is the equivalent of two fully loaded 747 jets plunging into the ocean every week for a year. It's 80 percent of the American death toll in Vietnam—only those losses spanned two decades, and in two decades we women have gone through sixteen Vietnams.

But again, the journey isn't a she thing. It's not a cancer thing. It's not intrinsic to life-threatening diseases, accidents or crimes, though they often spark a rapt search.

Something intrudes on the logical, linear progression of our lives, and we feel cheated. For me, it was the realization that the future wasn't going to deliver on my expectations, and my will had nothing to do with it.

Then I noticed this dandelion poking through a crack in the driveway and bursting into bloom. I saw my face in its flower. At first, I was reluctant to identify with a weed. But I realized it chose me.

Many months later, my life in a different circle, I was flipping through Anna Selby's gorgeous book, *Chinese Herbalism*, and found this story:

> The young daughter of a high official discovered a lump in her breast. This made her very frightened and ashamed. When her father found out about her condition, he became very angry, saying she must have done something immoral to have caused it. The girl pleaded her innocence but to deaf ears and, in despair, went to the river to take her life. As she jumped in, a fisherman and his daughter saw her and rescued her. The two girls were the same age and, as the fisherman's daughter gave her new friend dry clothes, she saw the reason for her despair. The fisherman said he knew of a herb to cure her, and over the following days she drank a liquid from the herb and applied a poultice of it to her breast. Her parents, filled with remorse, sought her out and were amazed to discover that she was cured. The fisherman gave her the herb

to continue to keep her well. She planted it in her garden and named it after the fisherman, whose name she never knew.[1]

The herb's name was dandelion.

The future brings us something different. Something more.

August 22, 1996

I remember: Riding fast up B Street, the sun at my back, the shadows long in front of me, pumping hard on Bill's old green bike.

If I held my arms tight at my side, I could erase the curves of my female body.

I looked stronger, more angular.

At 11: No hips. No boobs.

Now I see her again—on my empty left chest—with a drain dangling, a tube of blood leaving me.

Bones and muscles ache, as if emerging from a long hibernation.

Who has she come back to free, this half boy/prince?

August 23, 1996

I remember: In the shower, I would hear him waking, the insistent cries of a hungry baby, Big O. The boy who could suck nails out of a 2˝ by 4˝. That's how crazy he was to nurse.

"Anne, he goes forty-five minutes on each side. Is that enough?"

"Heck, yes. Cut him off after twenty. He doesn't need that much milk."

Owen ignored my sister's advice. He grew quickly, lusting to move, lusty for more.

So, in the shower I'd hear him, my hair full of lather.

"I'll be out in a couple of minutes, Paul. Hold him off."

But my nipples were hardening, poking forward and my breasts were tingling, more alive than I can ever remember. The milk spurted out like tiny fire hoses.

I grabbed them, pushing hard to stop the flow. "Let

---

1. From *Chinese Herbalism* by Anna Selby (Berkeley, CA: Ulysses Press, 1998), p. 92.

down," it's called. "Let out," it should be.

Then I would hurry out of the shower, scoop him
against my damp, naked body, my hair stuck against
my shoulders, and put my nipple into his mouth.

Oh, Owen, how you fed me.

I could not read the pathologist's report until recently. I would
stumble over unfamiliar words and wonder if there is anything funny
about "comedo-type" cells. I hoped so. But always I stuffed the report
back into the file before the question could rise: What did she do with
my breast?

After slicing the sections and slimming the ill-defined, tan-gray stuff
around, did she double bag it in plastic? Did it still look like a breast?
Was it burned that night?

I'm not really interested in hospital procedure. I'm wondering why
I didn't ask for it back. Why didn't I bury it in the backyard so I could
lay violets on it in the spring?

Violets: the forgiving flower, the ones that release their scent when
crushed.

But if I ask that question I will have to ask that other one, so heavily
guarded by shame. Why did I let my mother die alone, ravaged by a
virus, convulsing in a coma until her strong heart gave out? Why
weren't we there for her in the stretch, in the hospital room, braiding
her fingers into ours? We, who loved her so much. She, our North Star.

What was I protecting that was worth more than the comfort I
might have rendered?

Evening

The pathologist's findings determined my course of treatment. My cancer was classified a Stage 3. Prognosis *after* treatment: 50/50. This means I have a 50/50 chance of five-year survival.

My oncologist recommended a bone marrow transplant. I opted against it, not wanting to be away from Noah and Owen, then 7 and 10, for six to eight weeks. I also wasn't impressed by the 5 to 10 percent death rate during the procedure, and the lack of data showing long-term benefits.

I had twelve rounds of chemotherapy in nine months. Adriamycin first. It took out my hair and sterilized me. Instant menopause. It also made my heart beat at double time for a few days after treatment, engendering agitation and temporary despair. After two rounds I refused anymore. I then had six hits of Taxol and four of CMF.[1]

Six weeks into treatment I had a seizure in my doctor's office. The nurse was trying to flush the catheter implanted in my chest. The usual routine: heparin, saline, chemo. But she couldn't get an exchange. Pump, pump, pump. I tasted something funny, saw stars, heard strange music.

I guess I had a seizure. I felt something crashing back into the top of my head. I opened my eyes, or maybe I saw again through already open eyes. The nurses were studying me, worried. It lasted about a minute, they said.

My doctor suspected that cancer had spread to my brain, but the MRI that night showed only a bit of scarring. Could be an old injury, they said. The next day's EEG discovered a "left temporal lobe abnormality." No driving for six months and possibly a lifelong dependence on Dilantin, an antiseizure drug. The condition used to be called epilepsy.

---

1. CMF is a mixture of anticancer agents that consists of Cytoxan, methotrexate, and 5-fluorouracil.

Six weeks after that, the Port-a-cath broke—inside me. But nobody knew it.

On a Saturday night my heart began stopping, squeezing, lurching. Monday I called my oncologist's office. A nurse said that by the end of the week they might locate a Holter monitor to do diagnostic work on my heart. Meanwhile, two days later, I went in for chemo. My doctor heard the irregular beats, but wanted to proceed with chemo ("the medicine," as he called it, and I never could). Then a nurse had trouble with the port and suggested an x-ray.

That's when they saw the stub of the plastic line and found the rest floating in my heart. I was packed off to the hospital where a radiologist who specializes in angioplasty went in through a femoral vein in my thigh, snaked a tiny lasso into my heart and grabbed it. Had he not succeeded, I would have had open-heart surgery.

Five inches of white tubing: It could have accomplished what the cancer began—in a fraction of the time. Sweet tomorrow! I have the broken tubing in a baggie in the dining room, still coated with dried blood.

I didn't want another chest cath, so I got the next one implanted in my right arm. Ten weeks later, after playing basketball on a Friday night, I noticed my right arm was red and swollen. My hand puffy.

March 1, 1997, A.M.

> I believe my body is screaming in confusion, "Why, why do you keep doing this to me?" I don't have any good answers.

Another trip to the hospital, hours lying in the ER. A venogram confirmed clots in my subclavian vein. My immune system was attacking the tubing with phalanx after phalanx of platelets. And the platelets were falling, heaping up like gelatin.

March 1, 1997, P.M.

> From my fourth-floor window at Christ Hospital:
> Lightning trembles across the city. The sky turns purple.
> Thunder pounds (muffled by the air being blown into
> the room). Voices down the hall.
> Eight years ago, almost, I came here full of Noah,
> who eased gently into this world. What a sweet and

9

graceful boy! He was so still that snowy morning.
Confident in stillness.

Sometimes I think there must be something wrong
with me that I am not more moved by miracles. Was I
too aware of a full bladder or cramping womb to weep
for the life come out of me?

Tonight, alone with the favorite breast gone ("medical
waste"), my eggs killed by chemicals, my body in revolt
over a tube, I ask myself: At whose nativity have I been
summoned? Who will grow up out of my loins? Is there
a great work, a new child, a grace never before
expressed, heard, seen, or felt that I am here for?

I spent a couple days in the hospital getting high doses of heparin
intravenously to dissolve the clot. Then I began injecting myself at
home and finally swallowed the blood thinner, Coumadin, daily.

The dose required monitoring with frequent blood tests. Too little
Coumadin and the clots would regrow. Too much and I could bleed,
internally or externally. Brain hemorrhage a possibility.

Three weeks later my arm swelled again. Another venogram, another
occluded vein. Heart beating irregularly. Blood thinners boosted.

But my arm kept swelling. The clot was six inches long and growing
into my jugular vein. Spasms of pain shot through my head and inten-
sified. Narcotics could not dull it.

I settled things with Paul, my head locked in my arms, speaking slowly
through tears: A clean slate, thanks and love; go well with the boys.

The next day, a CT scan showed no cerebral bleeding, but the arm
cath was removed in a hurry. Headaches subsided. I survived it, though
I will remain on Coumadin indefinitely.

Final two rounds of chemo were injected in my left arm, despite the
precautions about never having an injection on the arm where so many
lymph nodes have been removed. In addition to the usual nausea,
fatigue, and constipation, I itched all over from a tiny red rash.

May 6, 1997

If the cancer returns, only then will I decide my next
move. And if people ask me that question now, I will
smack them down. Another example of nonuseful
thinking.

> Truth is, I don't want any more chemo. I don't want
> to do it again. I get nauseated thinking about it. I don't
> want the drugged stupor, the push of caustic chemicals
> handled by the gloved fingers of nurses—I am so tired
> of their needles. I can't think of a reason that this is
> good. Does it really work?

On that last day of treatment I went to my oncologist's office with a plate of cookies for the staff. In turn they gave me a coffee mug, decorated with their office logo and filled with Hershey kisses. They also gave me a gold-plated pin, courtesy of one of the drug companies, engraved with the words, "partnership for survival."

The attached card said the pin should be worn by everybody—doctors, nurses, researchers, pharmacists, hospital workers, family, friends and patients. "When you wear the partnership pin, you are not alone."

I got another infusion of chemicals that made my heart beat strangely again; the rash raged; the precious antinausea pills that cost $15 a piece could not quell the storm.

May 8, 1997

> My self-confidence, my life-confidence is shot. I'm
> just too depleted, too slow, too dull.

I would return to my oncologist two weeks later for a visit, following up on another bone scan, CT scan, MRI, EEG, x-ray, and mammogram. None detected globs of misguided cells.

He shook my hand and congratulated me on being cancer-free, and said my experience with chemotherapy was not typical. "Almost everything that could go wrong did."

I smiled with relief and a certain amount of survivor's guilt. I had actually avoided the mouth sores and infections that my friend Faye got and, for the moment, the lymphedema that was besieging another friend. But I also knew I was leaving those medical partners when my immune system was as vulnerable as it had ever been to any pathogen, including cancer.

No, I can't prove that, though I suspect there are markers in the blood revealing vitality or its lack. I just felt frail. I felt alone, and I needed more than a gold-plated pin.

But that was okay. I had a plan. I would gather my strength and go on another journey.

The Presence

I am here. All I need is here. It has always been here. It will always be here.

What is it?

Enough of everything I thought I didn't have enough of—money, time, knowledge, love. I even have solutions to problems that have not yet befallen me.

I have so much I won't go hungry. I know so much I can't be stumped or cheated. I am so well loved I don't fear rejection.

I share and am not depleted. I love freely.

I travel backward and forward and never run out of time.

Who, feeling such, believes?

A fool. A primitive. A mystic.

I wish I could.

Backward: In the summer of 1995, a year before I was diagnosed, we set out for Mt. Auburn Presbyterian Church on a hot, bright Sunday, more dressed down than usual. From church we were going to Cinergy Field to see the Reds play the Marlins. A neighbor had given us tickets for the blue seats. The best.

The boys and their cousin Will were bouncing around in the back seat, baseball caps already in place. "What's that light mean?" Paul asked, pointing to the dash.

The engine was overheating, the arrow on the temperature gauge flopping toward the right. We noticed clouds of smoke escaping from the hood and smelled something acrid. Paul pulled over, but before we could get out of the car, another driver in a pickup truck with a bicycle in the back pulled in front of us.

The tube between the radiator and the coolant tank had apparently snapped. There wasn't a single tool in our car. But the other guy had bike tools and strips of old rubber. He patched the line back together.

Our car needed more water. We didn't have any. He had a little left in his water bottle.

"This will get you to the nearest gas station," he said, and drove off.

He was right, though the nearest gas station was just a convenience store with gas pumps. We bought some coolant and decided to make a mad dash for home—about seven miles away.

Our car broke down again and again. Paul jogged back to the convenience store to call a tow truck, and the boys and I sat on the trunk of the car trying to persuade cousin Will that our other car worked.

Then, one by one, other cars stopped, their drivers offering help. The number was unbelievable. One car belonged to a family from our village, en route to grandma's house in Indiana. They insisted on turning around, squeezing us in and driving us home.

We missed church, but we were at the ballpark for the opening pitch. "We experienced our sermon," I told the boys as we squeezed into our seats.

Bad luck. Good luck. Goodwill.

A neat little package.

The memory lay like that, unchallenged, until the fall of 1996, a few months into cancer treatment. It was early morning, and I was riding on the bus to work. So much in my life had changed by then. I'd lost my breast, my hair, my fertility, and I'd had the seizure, which took care of driving privileges.

Yet in the stern gray of dawn, amid a crowd of strangers, I felt oddly good. It was more than that. I felt comforted, connected, supremely cared for. The sensation rippled up my spine and through my body. Even the rough-riding bus, which materialized out of darkness at the end of the street, seemed like a miracle.

What could account for this?

I had no answers. Instead, images of that car breakdown resurfaced, and I began asking myself whether "bad luck, good luck, goodwill" exhausted the possibilities. Those factors were all there. But what about the circumstances that had surrounded the bad luck—the fact that we were together, not me alone commuting to work? And what about the goodwill, which was timely, enthusiastic, and truly helpful?

Could there have been a Presence infusing the situation that was more attentive than I had imagined? Or maybe it had always been there, in every moment, and I was just becoming aware of it.

The desire is familiar enough. We'd probably all like to see the face of God, but would settle for assurances that God is around the corner, just out of sight.

I wanted—needed—to entertain that possibility of God's presence, but not with blind faith or intellectual laziness. Too many "believers" cultivate their faith on examples of the nice things that happen to them. Prosperity is a sign of finding favor with God. Somebody else's disease is an example of failure.

Rubbish, I said, although deep down I probably nursed a similar attitude.

But, really, could I make room in my life for an intimate Presence? What if I identified coincidences—synchronicities—that seemed remarkable? Could I celebrate them? Weave them into meaning?

And what about the bigger challenge: Could I see God in chaos? Perhaps my loss really wasn't one.

I was shivering with excitement.

Calamity

I see calamity now in every face I meet. Actually, I don't see it, but I know it's there.

It results from the breakup of a close relationship, the loss of a job, a serious disease, the death of a loved one. Each can catch us unprepared, shake us up, remind us of something we already know, but tend to ignore.

Life is a fatal condition, "a blood sport," as the late runner/doctor George Sheehan described it as prostate cancer bore down on him.

In one scene in the little picture book, *Buddhism for Sheep* by Chris Riddell, the sheep are gathered around a butcher shop window. They're staring at a sign announcing a special on lamb chops. Some look astonished. Others outraged. The caption reads: "It is necessary to gain the insight that life is impermanent." Why?

I think the correct answer is "detachment." But it is the scent of death that heightens my desire, making the more I want more desirable.

October 31, 1996

> It's so cliché, yet true: If this is my last Halloween, let it be memorable. Let me greet the children with enthusiasm. Let me feel the chill in the air, notice the stars and the candles burning inside pumpkins. Let me be amazed by the insects that flock to the light above our front door. I want to be fully present.

When calamity ripped the fabric of my life, I had no elegant prayers to patch it. All those churchgoing years, yet all I uttered was a simple plea, "God, be with me. Go with me."

I repeated it a lot, along with four words I said at the sight of every needle: "I can do this." I'm not phobic about injections. I don't mind the sharp sting. But I had to contend with ambivalent feelings about cancer treatment, and "I can do this" cut the unknown into manageable pieces.

It also put me in dialogue with myself.

Every morning, from the bus stop to work five blocks away, I sang Tallis's Canon I had heard so often in church: "Go with us Lord and light the way, through this and every coming day. That with thy spirit strong and true, our lives may be our gift to you." I can't explain why it clarified that sense of a Presence and seemed to carry me beyond danger. I just know that it did.

Tuesday, December 3, 1996

> My eyes are like fish tanks, full of water. My heart
> squeezes, oddly, randomly within my chest. I am afraid.
> All morning I have fought it off—fear and dizziness,
> sweaty palms, sweat creeping up the back of my
> neck—trying to keep my mind focused, trying to look
> ahead.

I did not know then that the crazed heartbeats were caused by the broken catheter. I'd been coexisting with five inches of tubing in my heart, running and working, for four days and would do so for another day before the problem was identified and addressed.

There were moments when death felt near. One occurred during an Xavier basketball game after we walked up three flights of steps to find our seats. As the boys dashed ahead, I pulled Paul aside and reminded him where to find my will and insurance policies. Then we sat down and made it through half of the game.

I was afraid, but I kept thinking of a beloved aunt and uncle who were coming to see us the next day. I didn't want to miss them, and I didn't want to be in a hospital.

There is fear, and then there is fear of fear. Because of the latter, I delayed action on the former. I prayed and sang quietly instead. On the bus to work Tuesday, with my left hand covering my notebook, I explicated each line of Tallis's Canon, searching for intimations of immortality.

Words are clunky things, inexact and often callused into uselessness. But they amble with us down pathways. They transport us into our past. They bump into hopes and occasionally stumble onto a mine of private images, emotions, meaning.

Lisel Mueller has a poem called "When I Am Asked" about how—
or why, really—she ventured into poetry. She tells it far better, in fewer
words, the day after her mother died, going into a beautiful garden and
being unable to dialogue with flowers.

> I sat on a gray stone bench
>
> ringed with the ingenue faces
>
> of pink and white impatiens
>
> and placed my grief
>
> in the mouth of language,
>
> the only thing that would grieve with me.[1]

Sometimes after writing a lot I find myself in the middle of a mis-
spelled word, often a homonym, and while I'm scratching it out, grateful that no one will see my foolish mistake, I realize that while wrong,
the word hinted at a bigger right.

I turn and confront something I'd never noticed. I see with
improved sight.

This is what dreams do, I'm convinced of it. They're stocked with
puns and *trompe l'oeils,* associations more clever than we are. They tease
us to untangle them. But, like prayers, we shrug them off.

Dreams, how strange; prayers, how wishful.

I confess it: My nights have been full of dreams, my days of those
sort-of prayers. I began to look at almost every event as significant, and
I have yet to be disappointed. This may be a sneaky universe, but it's
not loaded with superfluity.

One morning I stopped on the way home from an early run, hat
pulled tight over my bald head. I look around. It was as if a voice
hailed me.

November 12, 1996

> I realized I needed to linger a bit with the stars and
> the clouds of dawn. Suppose they have something to
> say to me, could I hear it? Have I waited, no matter the

---

1. Reprinted by permission of Louisiana State University Press from *Alive Together:
New and Selected Poems,* by Lisel Mueller, p. 198. Copyright © 1986, 1991,
1992, 1994, 1995, 1996 by Lisel Mueller. Originally published in *Waving From
Shore: Poems,* copyright © 1986 by Lisel Mueller. Used by permission.

circumstances, for that message? Can I understand the broader sense of connection?

About an hour later, after walking the boys to school, I was met by a neighbor. She came out of her house and grabbed me by the collar. I laughed with uncertainty. She is an accomplished writer, but that's all I knew of her. "Come in, I have something for you," she said.

It was a poem by Robert Francis called "Summons." I shook my head as I read it:

> Keep me from going to sleep too soon
> Or if I go to sleep too soon
> Come wake me up. Come any hour
> Of night. Come whistling up the road.
> Stomp on the porch. Bang on the door.
> Make me get out of bed and come
> And let you in and light a light.
> Tell me the northern lights are on
> And make me look. Or tell me clouds
> Are doing something to the moon
> They never did before, and show me.
> See that I see. Talk to me till
> I'm half awake as you
> And start to dress wondering why
> I ever went to bed at all.
> Tell me the walking is superb.
> Not only tell me but persuade me.
> You know I'm not too hard persuaded.[2]

Seventeen months later I find myself sitting with her in a tiny restaurant where I've never been before. She with butterscotch eyes, keen mind, and self-deprecating laugh. Me with hair so thick it must be thinned every six weeks. We are huddled over grilled cheese and tuna salad, discussing words as if they were a huge, unexpected inheritance.

---

2. From Robert Francis' *Collected Poems: 1936–1976* (Amherst, MA: University of Massachusetts Press, 1976), p. 149. Copyright by Robert Francis. Used with permission.

Outside a March wind is snapping awnings, stirring the dirt in the gutters. I look around the restaurant, blessing its bins of coffee beans, its chalkboard with the day's specials in colored chalk, its displays of rich desserts.

The clouds of dawn, so many months ago: Was this their message? That conspiring Presence: Was this its gift?

Presents

Backward still: Before I watched for the Presence, there were presents. Casseroles, phone calls, flowers, Robin's bread, cassettes from Megan and Sarah, books and more books, weekly cards from Jerry. They amazed me, connecting me to a community where I seemed to occupy the village green.

Ten days after diagnosis, I documented that day's mail: a Furrows flier, a booklet of coupons, a Sears flier, a packet of campaign materials from the Leukemia Society, one shareholder's report, one letter of solicitation, a performance contract for Paul, and twenty-one cards and letters of encouragement for me.

August 29, 1996

Twenty-one! This too is nirvana.

Doesn't every person with a life-threatening condition talk of this?

August 30, 1996

Gifts keep rolling in. It's sort of like experiencing one's own funeral, only with the potential of being resurrected by it.

I felt as if I was lying back in a bed of arms, cradled and cooed over. I've never been in a mosh pit, but perhaps the experience is similar. A couple months later I described it as giving "a jolt of joy so potent it seemed capable of rewiring my brain."

If it had succeeded, how would I be different?

I would live out of gratitude and receptivity, and it wouldn't matter for how long. That's what I tried to tell my oncologist the first time we met: "How can I want more?" We were talking about the amount of time different treatments might supply. He looked puzzled. "I think after two years you will surely want more time."

He was right. But I was not wrong.

Gratitude is a very sturdy dwelling. It withstands weather, human capriciousness, and those so-called acts of God, which aren't. But it's a magical state, authentic or nothing at all.

Somehow, though I can't explain it, receptivity is its close neighbor. I visited there, in brief and golden moments, letting myself go, releasing my judgments.

But I couldn't remain in that open state because I felt I didn't deserve its grace. I would see Betsy in her apron, cutting her trophy flowers for me, handing me a plate of cookies with yellow frosting faces.

My words of thanks began to sound hollow to me. I knew I shouldn't be measuring all that came to me against my worth. But I couldn't help it.

September 12, 1996

I am closing the door. The front door. The bedroom door. I am unplugging the phone. I am crawling into bed to escape, regroup, complain. Another bottom is falling out. This is the one that holds up the public face, the cheerful acceptance. This is the one that does the dancing monkey routine.

I've been gagging on self-help, how-to, inspirational, and educational books—enough of life's real edges, real decisions. Enough of being sick. Of taking. Of having so much handed to me that I feel overwhelmed, as if I can't be cranky or mean-spirited anymore, ever, in my life.

I would joke about that afternoon when I went to my room with a randy work of fiction and took a long nap. It seemed like an act of rebellion—necessary, but adolescent. I thought I was just tired, indulging in a detour. Tomorrow I would get back to gratitude. I would try harder.

I didn't know that it wasn't a detour. Sometimes the way to move ahead is to travel back, to give unworthiness its voice and shame a place where it doesn't have to blush. I didn't know that in silencing those feelings I was sabotaging my life.

Knowing

Faye knew my diagnosis before I did. She knew it even before the surgeon or the pathologist.

I don't know how she knew. But when I spotted her at church on Sunday before the Monday morning biopsy, she did not smile. Her look was direct, dark, unspeakably sad. I turned away, shook my head in our pew, and mumbled to myself:

"She doesn't get it. This is nothing. My obstetrician said it was nothing. The surgeon said it was nothing. He said, 'I've felt a lot of cancer in my time and this doesn't feel like cancer.' For heaven's sake, he's gray-haired and balding; 'my time' must be about thirty years."

Only now do I understand how much Faye wanted to be wrong. She didn't know my diagnosis. All she knew is that a breast biopsy is not something you face with either denial or an "atta-girl" grin.

She's been there—in the operating suite, the rooms where bone scans, CT scans, and MRIs are made. She's held out her right arm and her left arm for needles. She's waited for tests and wilted at their results. She's taken poison and retched her guts out.

Faye has had breast cancer twice.

She's still in the cycle of testing every three months. She's had red flags and false alarms and little bumps on her skin that had to come off. Yet she lives well, managing a more-than-full-time job as an editor and educator. She is a wife, mother, and swooning grandmother. Tough, funny, devoted. She is a person who is trying to keep fear in its place.

"I wanted to phone you this morning," she wrote me the day of my mastectomy, "but I suspect you've received so many calls that you need no more. However, I prayed for your hormone receptors and lymph nodes, for that small piece of absolute terror that is lodged somewhere in your being, for your ability to remain focused and in control, yet open and vulnerable enough to receive the love and healing that comes from God through other people."

A few days after the surgery, when all the tests results were in and my future charted, we met in Ault Park, sipped coffee and ate muffins. She handed me a bag of articles and a cloth prosthesis that she had worn.

I was still bandaged, so I nested it in my hands. The human breast is as varied in size and shape as the bodies of jellyfish. Yet this soft mound of spun fibers was a perfect match.

"You don't have to give it back. I'm never going to use it again," she said.

Somewhere along the way she figured out that she could live without breasts—real ones, cloth ones, or silicone ones. She could also shrug at people who might want to stare. Among other things, her flat chest is a silent sermon to a culture that undervalues the wonder of breasts and overvalues their decorative appeal.

This is not to say she didn't grieve over their loss. I can only imagine how much.

But none of Faye's phone calls and letters made me pity her. Or me. In the words she wrote I heard her voice, with its distinctive Kentucky wash. Her handwriting, erect as a ladder-back chair, reminded me of her teacherly disciplines. Her coping techniques clued me to a wild streak.

This encouraged me to dig down and release my own, never knowing how much disappointment is assuaged by the silly or the bold.

A close friend of hers, actually a minister, suggested she tell me "how much joy I received during chemo from shouting the word *f—*. I must confess that it did offer some type of calming quality to my state. I really don't believe that particular word was in my repertoire of exclamations prior to chemo."

Faye recommended lots of hand washing and no shared food. Avoid the kids' library books. Buy only cotton scarves and hats; other fabrics fall off a bald head. Challenge the "ole boys' club" (i.e., doctors). Look for reasons to laugh.

Actually, she never said that one. She just signed nearly every letter with words of wisdom that got the corners of my mouth moving in the right direction. A sampling:

"I think animal testing is a terrible idea. They get all nervous and give the wrong answers."

"If a woman has to choose between catching a fly ball and saving an infant's life, she'll choose to save the infant's life, without even considering if there are men on base."

"The hypothalamus is one of the most important parts of the brain involved in many kinds of motivation. Among other functions, the hypothalamus controls the 'four F's': (1) fighting (2) fleeing (3) feeding (4) mating.*"

"Madness takes its toll. Please have exact change."

"Experience is that marvelous thing that enables you to recognize a mistake when you make it again."

"Kermit the Frog: 'Time's fun, when you're having flies.' "

"As always, forgive spelling. I do windows and floors, but not spelling. Love you, Faye."

---

* Word has been changed.

Listening

When Kay called and invited me to join the group, I said thanks. Sounds good, but I'm too busy, I'm always tired and I can't get there. I'd just had the seizure and wasn't allowed to drive.

I had been trying to be less dependent on other people, but now I needed more assistance. Alternate transportation everywhere.

Back in August when I was diagnosed, my friend and neighbor Betsy issued a blanket invitation to watch our boys whenever I needed to go to doctors' appointments. But how many times could I keep turning to her or, when Paul was busy, asking her husband, Buz, or our minister, Hal, or other friends for rides? I was afraid of wearing out my welcome.

Their generosity was almost a burden. The sense of I-don't-deserve-this was gnawing at me, like a mouse on a cereal box. I kept measuring their goodness against a buried, unexpressed feeling of inadequacy.

Yet Kay's offer intrigued me.

Sensing my interest and convinced of the merits of the experiment, she would not be dissuaded easily. "We'll pick the best time for you," she said, "and find a way to get you here, if you want to come."

Well, okay. I'd try a few sessions. But I'd ask Paul for help first.

"What is 'this group'?" he asked that night. "And who's Kay?"

Kay's name isn't Kay. But she is a woman I'd met a decade earlier in some journalistic capacity. Her life had changed; she'd become the marketing director of a holistic health center. She wasn't calling to promote the center. It was to let me in on a pilot project. Something the medical director had wanted to try for a long time: Group therapy for women with breast cancer.

He believed the empathy of a group creates powerful medicine—something greater than the sum of the ingredients.

Support groups for cancer patients aren't a novel idea. They comprise the cornerstone of Wellness Community programs, and they've been offered by various other nonprofits for years. But, in the case of breast cancer, the medical value of such groups has been championed by a professor of psychiatry at Stanford University, Dr. David Spiegel.

Spiegel's much-cited research involved eighty-six women whose cancer had spread beyond the breast. The chances of remission were slim, their prognoses poor.

Although he set up his 1976 research scientifically, randomly designating some women for the experimental group and others for no group, he wasn't looking for data that would impress scientists. He simply hoped to show that the character of a patient's life could be enriched and death "detoxified."

It was almost by accident, nearly a decade later, he discovered that the women in the group hadn't just lived better. They'd lived longer. On average, eighteen months longer than women in the control group.

Had he been testing a new drug, such results would have been heralded by cancer specialists. Anything that can extend life expectancy by thirty percent is called significant. Yet what an unassuming nostrum he offered—a weekly opportunity to look at fear, express longings, dignify one's dying.

Spiegel and other researchers have replicated the original experiment, not just with breast or other cancer patients, but people with AIDS and heart disease. They're also assaying the blood in ways they didn't dream of before, trying to identify the markers of a thriving spirit.

But already Spiegel is convinced: Group support is essential, he says. Cancer specialists who omit it are committing malpractice.

Thousands of women in Cincinnati have breast cancer, but only two women were waiting in the office of the doctor, whom I'll call The Listener, when I walked in for the first two-hour meeting in November of 1996.

Our common link was a disease that threatened to kill us in midlife. To them, I probably seemed strangely accepting. If I was angry or fearful about the disease, those emotions were deeply buried.

Sunday, November 24, 1996

> (The Listener) talked about the nature of cells, their
> electrical fields, the intelligence of the immune system—
> how it receives information and orchestrates elaborate
> processes—and the possibility of improving communi-

cation between the cells. He described cancer cells as
normal cells that are no longer fulfilling their destiny to
function normally. He talked of the need to communicate
with them, to help them become, to love them.

Thinking back, I realize I don't know much more about The
Listener now than I learned then. I don't know his age, where he went
to school, who influenced his career, or how he could possibly suggest
loving the cells that everyone was hell-bent on destroying. I know that
he was a neurologist who retrained in psychiatry, recognizing the
dynamic interchange between mind and body.

Over time others have told me he is highly respected by his peers.

But counseling relationships are not reciprocal. They don't grow on
swapped information, on mutual revelations of hurts and hopes.
Unused to such arrangements, I didn't like it at first. I felt too exposed.

Something has changed my opinion. I appreciate the relationship's
clear boundaries and absence of expectations. I hear myself telling
people I am alive because of psychotherapy.

Does that mean I didn't need surgery? didn't benefit from chemotherapy?

How could I make such a claim? I can't see into my own cells. But
I see now that I needed more than a surgeon and an oncologist could
provide. I respect and like each of those specialists and know they
worked hard for me.

But cancer gave me an opportunity to take on much more than
cancer. Perhaps that's because I was confused, itching, unknowingly,
for change. Perhaps that was its gift.

Cancer gave me thoughts that ruined sleep. It made my heart ache
so hard I couldn't ignore it. It brought the stars down to talk in my
ears. It forced Paul and me to start growing up with each other.

I'm not talking about merely extending existence. There are probably
millions of hack doctors who can and do keep people going and are
reimbursed handsomely for it. But how many can suggest a path through
our own deep woods to a clearing where the light shines down? How
many know that it is precious to find it?

The theologian Paul Tillich wrote, "Sometimes it happens that we
receive the power to say 'yes' to ourselves, that peace enters into us and

makes us whole, that self-hate and self-contempt disappear, and that our self is reunited with itself. Then we say that grace has come upon us."[1]

On January 3, 1997, one of the women couldn't make it to the session. By now The Listener had closed his second downtown office and had moved into the holistic center across town. It's an old Tudor-style mansion with high ceilings, dark wood, stained glass and leaded glass, Rookwood hearths, and windows that must be cranked by hand. The center feels far removed from Cincinnati, though the city surrounds it.

I was comfortable with the group, but I picked through my thoughts, selected my words. I could control emotion that way. Or so I thought.

Sunday, January 4, 1997

> A powerful session yesterday. I don't remember when I began to weep. It was something (she) was saying that revealed to me how punishing I feel this whole regimen of chemotherapy is. My eyes were closed and I was weeping and saying that I was surviving because I am fighting it (the treatment) off. I could never connect with chemo being a good thing.

The difficulty of treatment was convincing me that I must have done something wrong, something that brought on cancer and then those bizarre complications. The sense that I was undergoing punishment stirred a fear that may be older than I am, encoded on another mutant gene, whispering that I hadn't just done wrong; I was wrong.

From original sin, it's a short hike into hopelessness.

I hadn't realized I was short on hope. Or that my recovery may have been undermined by self-judgment. But even if I had known it, or someone had revealed it to me like another damn diagnosis, I could not have willed it away.

What mattered was that afternoon I witnessed a private truth. Then I clothed an orphaned feeling with words.

How many more changelings are out there, I wondered, shivering in the orbit of me?

---

1. From *The Shaking of the Foundation* by Paul Tillich (New York: Charles Scribner's Sons, 1948), p. 163.

My mind, urged on by a disquieted heart, began running in reverse, leapfrogging into my childhood, asking questions I'd shrunk from before. The past had seemed irrelevant. Only people who like to wallow go there, I believed. Slurp, slurp, slurp. I could hear their boots sinking into the mud.

But in the weeks and months that followed, my journals became trail maps, full of squiggly lines, arrows, and ellipses.

It's like that Indiana Jones game Noah plays on the computer. Indy walks through a one-way door into a stone chamber. He's searching for a hidden staircase, a moving wall or Roman amphora—anything that will help him get out of the chamber.

Each accomplishment begets another challenge, concealing another lesson. On and on he goes, forward and backward, a little closer to the ark or the grail, though he can never be sure.

No wonder the history of the human soul is depicted in epics. That's how it feels to travel toward consciousness—baffling, adventurous, and awfully repetitive.

"I had imagined that the loss of a breast would create catharsis, that I would emerge like a phoenix from the fire, reborn, with all things made new, especially the pain in my heart," wrote poet/novelist May Sarton in June of 1979, after her cancer-filled left breast was removed.[2]

"I had imagined that real pain, physical pain and physical loss would take the place of mental anguish and the loss of love. Not so. It has all to be begun again, the long, excruciating journey through pain and rejection, through anger and not understanding, toward some regained sense of my self."

"Watch your dreams," The Listener said, as I walked out of the room that day. I nodded, though it took me many months to learn how to watch, how to catch, how to extrapolate from the images and emotions of sleep. But it didn't take me long to notice I wasn't quite the same.

The next week I smiled shyly as I reported to the group: *"For the first time, I feel hope."* They clapped and hooted.

I had begun another journey—the one that will lead me Home.

---

2. From *Recovering: A Journal* by May Sarton, p. 119. Copyright © 1980 by May Sarton. Reprinted by permission of W. W. Norton & Company, Inc.

Sleep

All creatures—mammals, reptiles, and insects—need sleep, according to the boys' encyclopedia, *The New Book of Knowledge*, which is a bit older than newer. "Without a period of rest following periods of activity, the mind and body would become too fatigued to work properly."

"Comparatively little is known about what causes a person to fall asleep and what causes a person to stay awake. There are many theories, but no single theory is accepted by all scientists. Some believe that the day's activities use up a 'wakefulness' substance stored in the brain, which is then renewed during sleep."[1]

The person who trotted out this theory has not, perhaps, experienced the inconstancies of sleep, which seem to be based on needs other than renewal.

I end a trying day at the usual time, but with an unusual desire for sleep. My "wakefulness substance" feels as though it has been sucked, squeezed, drained. Sleep takes over quickly. But within two or three hours this life-giving state of unconsciousness evaporates and in its place sits a thought, heavy-hipped, or perhaps three of them bickering.

I try to be patient. Think one thought through. Think another. Consider the alternative. Yes but. This isn't fair. I really don't care. I want to sleep. So peaceful, I lie to myself. No more thoughts. Nighty-night. . . . Oh, please. I have to get up at 6:00. So much I have to do. I need this sleep.

That's garden-variety insomnia trying to argue a thought out of its power. The NFL linebacker version comes with calamity, when you know all bargaining will be for naught.

---

1. From *The New Book of Knowledge*, vol. 17 (Danbury, CT: Grolier Books, 1991), p. 201. Copyright © 1991 by Grolier Incorporated.

August 20, 1996, 12:15 a.m.

> I wish I could sleep. My head is a fat knot of fatigue.
> But also a fat knot of thoughts. I feel icky, not terrible,
> just icky. That haunting spiritual keeps playing in my
> head, "Sometimes I feel like a motherless child." I think
> of myself at nineteen, too young to lose my mother. I
> think of Elizabeth, Caitlin, and Will at ten, eight, and
> six, too young to lose their father.

I didn't write about what I was obviously thinking, Owen and Noah. They were too young to lose their mother. And I, too, felt unready. Underexpressed.

I didn't know about how Paul would manage. I was too caught up in myself.

I got out of bed, inched down the dark stairs, and positioned myself on the couch. Just one light on. A Bible across my lap. Hal, our minister, had suggested I "work with" the Twenty-third Psalm. To me, "work with" means rewrite it—create a setting for it to play out its drama. Line by line, word by word.

The exercise reminded me of college, picking apart one of Gerard Manley Hopkins's poems, trying to balance its meaning like a broom on my fingertip. "I caught this morning morning's minion, kingdom of daylight's dauphin, dapple-dawn-drawn Falcon."

How many good walks I have had with Hopkins, just trying to tongue his words, let alone understand them. How many values I owe to Wordsworth. How much I would like to ask Emily Dickinson about all the words she capitalizes in her poems. "Why?"

But I think I'd be intimidated by her stare. After all, she stood alone, on behalf of herself, when critics told her she should demure to lower case.

But back to the Bible: I know little of the lives of sheep. All I know is what I saw at seventeen outside Halsey, Oregon, the town where my brother lived briefly. What I saw was slaughter. One day I took his two dogs out with me while I rode his bike through the flat Willamette Valley. The dogs took off, leaped into a farmer's field, and attacked the sheep.

It was early spring. The lamb's blood seemed brighter against the green grass. Horribly so.

In spite of that, or maybe because of it, the Twenty-third Psalm did good things for me. Suppose a shepherd had been there that afternoon. Would the dogs have tasted fresh lamb?

When I translated the psalm, it evoked the Presence:

> God is my treasured friend. I am never alone.
>
> God goes with me into green fields, hikes with me along rivers, swims with me in Lake Huron, refreshes my soul.
>
> God opens the path for me and ventures with me into pine forests.
>
> Even though disease is a reality and death a possibility, God reaches out for me, holds my hand, keeps fear away; I do find comfort.
>
> When circumstances overwhelm, when communication is blocked, when the world is full of strangers: Even then I feel You working for me, taking care of my needs, conspiring for my fulfillment.
>
> Surely there is no greater joy than to experience your mercy and charity each day of my life.

That which I call the Presence gave me the courage to be alone and awake when I thought I needed to be asleep at someone's side. It was with me when the rules of my life began to change, when writing became not a professional activity, but a lifeline.

One night Paul heard sounds and came downstairs, blinking in the light, surprised to see me up "at that hour" (Isn't that how parents make the night taboo?) with a journal across my lap.

"Is something wrong?" he asked.

"No," I answered, though I could have said, "Yes. Everything."

But by the time I rethought my words, he had disappeared into the darkness, and I returned to my search.

I would never brag that I solved the problem of insomnia. First, because I'm reluctant to call it a problem any more and second, because it really could become a problem. Don't fence life into my expectations: That is one of the few absolutes I remind myself to live with.

But sleeplessness is easier. I've quit resisting it. For months I got up and wrote or read when it occurred. Or I propped up in bed and meditated.

It wasn't a nightly thing, but it happened enough that I felt tired a lot. I didn't like it. And not liking it was another form of resistance.

Then, I changed the message. To the surging feelings, the tangled thoughts I said, "Welcome. Talk to me. Teach me." One night I felt a jolt in my heart, as if a stake were being pounded. Other nights my feet tingled and twitched. My chest felt like a coffin, six inches long, three inches wide with screws at every corner.

I don't seem to be adept at visualization, at least not when I try to be. So I would just cover my heart with a hand. I would promise all the accusations that they'd get a fair hearing. They wouldn't have to wait until morning.

But oddly, once I gave in, they became courteous. They shook me and subsided.

In 1918, during a night of tortuous sleep and exhausting dreaming, Swiss novelist Hermann Hesse tried to listen to two different inner voices. One told him to ignore his feelings of sorrow, to go on, overcome his suffering. The other told him not to run, but to go right up to it.

"Love your suffering," this voice counseled. "Do not resist it, do not flee from it. Taste how sweet it is in its essence, give yourself to it, do not meet it with aversion. It is only your aversion that hurts, nothing else. Sorrow is not sorrow, death is not death if you do not make them so! Suffering is magnificent music—the moment you give ear to it. But you never listen to it; you always have a different, private, stubborn music and melody in your ear which you will not relinquish and with which the music of suffering will not harmonize."[2]

Hesse decided that neither voice is all wrong or all right. They're part of a duet that gets played through time, the volume, rhythm, and melody changing. But he was clearly drawn to the voice willing to

---

2. From *My Belief: Essays on Life and Art* by Hermann Hesse (New York: Farrar, Strauss and Giroux, 1974), p. 53. Translation copyright © 1974 by Farrar, Strauss and Giroux, Inc.

entertain the unwanted voice of sorrow. Perhaps he sensed what the-ologian Martin Buber would declare: "All suffering prepares the soul for vision."

It profits little, the experts say, to try to figure out why you got cancer. When you get your why, you can't roll it into a pill and swallow it. It won't give you any life. It probably won't even bring you much peace.

But the mind and conscience go their own way. At least mine have, fueled by energies and impulses, longings and regrets. Why should I wish to banish them? It's like those other questions, Why would I want to kill the messenger that disease is?

Why would I deny death its marvelous intelligence?

February 28, 1997

In the night when doubts descended, I heard a voice within me say, "Wait, why don't you go there? I love you." Is this the voice of God I wish to hear? Oh, probably. Just a piece of myself. Nothing more. But it put me back to sleep and in the morning I decided, "This is the beginning of faith." It comes not from will, but from letting go . . . to intuition, to God, to the amazing Presence, which keeps revealing itself.

Grounding

A few weeks ago I bumped into Bob, an acquaintance I had not seen in years. "What are you doing these days?" he asked.

I wondered if I looked different, older, more haggard than in his memory. I also paused as I do when asked this question. I don't like to be pushed to parade my efforts for smiles or frowns.

"I've come through breast cancer," I said. "I'm writing about healing."

Although a smile played across his face, his eyes seemed to grab at me. "Would that be traditional or holistic, much of which is more traditional than what we call traditional. Allopathic, homeopathic, ayurvedic? Are we talking psychic healing, faith healing, the use of prayer, breathing, body work, energy work—in this city, in the country, the world?"

His encyclopedic question silenced me. He obviously knew more than I did. I felt the despair that used to grip my stomach as a young reporter and grips it still in certain dreams. I'm not ready. I don't know enough. I never will know enough.

On my first job in Indiana, I was sent to Ohio to cover a court case and rushed back with the story, quoting the ruling of the "common police judge." It seemed fitting for a story about a town official found guilty of embezzlement. I didn't know the court's title is "common pleas." I merely wrote what my ears heard, and I burned when I was corrected.

The heat began to rise again into the sprockets of my brain that turn, but don't catch. I haven't read enough, researched enough, experienced enough. I shouldn't be doing this.

Beneath the fear of inadequacy lies a fear of authority and a vague expectation that all my shortcomings will bring forth the Executioner: "Into the fire, you stupid wench."

I've tried traditional and nontraditional medicine. I've started new treatments with all the hopes for perfection that one brings to marriage or the birth of a child.

I've been a good patient and a difficult patient and a better one for being difficult.

I don't know a lot. But I know what Bob never will know—my heart and my heartburn, my confusion, insomnia and desperate prayers, my morning runs and afternoon meditations, my fleeting moments of triumph when understanding has burst on me like an unexpected friend with a bag of apples.

He has not lain loving hands on my inadequacies. I have.

"It's a mishmash," I told him, my right toe making circles on the carpeting. "I'm just writing about what works for me."

Despite that epiphany or whatever it was with Bob, I still felt I needed to go to a lecture a few nights later, when a doctor talked of using alternative therapies at his family practice clinic. I'd heard enthusiastic reports from a number of patients, and I thought that perhaps he would reveal the essence of healing. Maybe, I thought, it involves some technique I haven't tried.

He dimmed the lights and clicked through a carousel of slides, many of which were just words on a blue background. The standard pedagogical approach. Poker face. Passion-free.

A few pictures that he'd taken of a psychic surgeon in the Philippines were impressive. The practitioner's fingers were pulling out stomach acids and infected tissue without making any incisions. The lecturing doctor didn't offer any explanations about how a wall of skin could be penetrated by unseen forces or why pain wasn't an issue or how diseased tissue could emerge intact.

Such speculation may have seemed unscientific in that gathering. You never know when a spy from the AMA might be in attendance. Every treatment and every herb that he mentioned "needs to be verified by the same standards that we verify conventional medicine," he said.

This means research funding, double-blind studies, validity based on a preponderance of statistical evidence. Yes, I know this is necessary for ingested substances. It's a reasonable expectation for anything that purports to fix or cure.

But it means taking a healing art and standardizing it into a commodity, giving it a slot in a protocol and a number on a reimbursement schedule. What works in Kansas City must work in Bangor, Maine. Cookbook medicine.

What will managed care do with prayer?

When he spoke of placebo effects, which he said can account for a third of cures, it was with a note of disdain. Would a person who has recovered, inexplicably, from Stage four pancreatic cancer share his disdain, I wondered.

He said nothing about the interaction between the one who comes for healing and the one who attempts to pass it along, nothing about entering a sacred space or sharing an intention.

November 8, 1996

> Yesterday I went with Estelle to St. Francis DeSales Church where those sweet nuns, Alice and Mary Ann, had arranged a blessing service with Father Ed, Brother John, and Kathy. Sweet is the word, again, that comes to me. The rose in a vase, the candle burning on a simple low table, the ritualized prayer, the ointment on my forehead and hands—mostly these hands touching me, one by one. My eyes pooled in gratitude. They almost do again. The intentionality made it beautiful and powerful. I am trying to hold that sweetness in the face of other demons.

Diane Ackerman, author of *A Slender Thread*,[1] tells of her stint as a phone counselor in a crisis- and suicide-prevention center in an interview. "It's very frustrating when you hear someone suffering. You wish you could befriend them, but that's taboo. The most you can do is listen athletically, hearing the words, the sighs, all the diphthongs of grief. Listening can be a life-giving act. Confiding strengthens the immune system."

I'm not sure how someone can know that. But I know that when I trust enough to speak my secrets and am met with receptivity, shackles are broken. The power of such moments spreads warmth from my heart through my body.

---

1. Diane Ackerman, *A Slender Thread: Rediscovering Hope at the Heart of Crisis* (New York: Vintage Books, 1998). Copyright © 1997 by Diane Ackerman.

A good listener needs to give no answers, only the breathing silence that dignifies the question.

Elie Wiesel notes that "a Hasidic tradition tells us that in the Torah the white spaces, too, are God-given."[2] So it is in the patient silence connecting speaker and listener.

But the lecturer spoke nothing of that. His talk, followed by a question-and-answer period stretched over two hours. I drank cups of water from the table in the back, but my imagination felt parched. I had wanted that giddy humility engendered by things obscure and wonderful.

I left disappointed, though not entirely empty-handed.

He said something I had experienced—a way of distinguishing holistic treatments from conventional ones: "The focus of traditional medicine is to decrease disease. The focus of a lot of alternative therapies is geared to increasing life force."

It was terse, yet striking. Maybe these practices need each other, though in ways peculiar to each person. His words helped me understand why chemotherapy had left me hungry and tired, and yet for other people, like Faye, chemotherapy could sometimes feel like a "stream of life," as she put it.

Later his words provided me with a test for measuring medical practitioners. No matter what the shingle says, no matter whether conventional or unconventional, no matter the magazines in the waiting room, is this person more interested in chasing pathology or building health? One makes my brain hot and tired. The other loosens my bones and lengthens my stride.

Looking back over treatment, I know I needed more chi. The uncharted parts of me needed more knowing, more poetry. They still do.

"No place," says novelist Wallace Stegner, "not even a wild place, is a place until it has had that human attention that at its highest reach we call poetry."[3]

---

2. From *All Rivers Run to the Sea* by Elie Wiesel, p. 321. Copyright © 1995 by Alfred A. Knopf, Inc. Reprinted by permission of the publisher.
3. From *Where the Bluebird Sings to the Lemonade Springs: Living and Writing in the West* by Wallace Stegner (New York: Penguin Books, 1992), p. 205. Copyright © 1992 by Wallace Stegner.

Wonders

Twenty years ago I gave my dad Ivan Illich's book *Medical Nemesis.* I don't know why. I only flipped through it in the bookstore, but it looked challenging in ways Daddy likes to be challenged. I don't know whether he ever read it, but when he deposited it on the toss-out pile about five years ago, I took it home, put it on a shelf, and forgot about it. Six months ago Paul pulled it off.

"Camilla, I think you ought to take a look at this book."

"Huh?"

"I think you'd like it."

Silence. My mind was someplace else.

I discovered it several weeks later on the back of the toilet. I flipped it open and read. My hands began to burn.

The holistic health movement was in its infancy when Illich began researching this brazen, meticulously documented book, published in 1976. Even the term *holistic* was only on the edges of parlance.

Illich set out to challenge the "progress" of conventional, modern medicine—an act as heretical as defaming motherhood and apple pie. He didn't advocate "holistic" health; he didn't even mention it. Nor did he envision the growth of alternative treatments, which is now accelerating into the mainstream. If he promoted anything, it was personal responsibility, "self-care among the laity," as he tamely put it.

Yet his thinking helped anchor the pilings on which the holistic health movement has been built.

I have an image of this irate social philosopher stomping his foot, waving his arms, and pointing to stacks of research studies, as if saying, "You're not as smart as we think you are. You hinder as often as you help. You don't even know the essentials of healing."

Such is the force of his words.

Illich develops his argument around the assertion that "a vast amount of contemporary clinical care is incidental to the curing of disease."[1] He also details a host of doctor-induced or treatment-induced illnesses, which have escalated costs and spawned new woes.

Although he acknowledges that antibiotics and vaccines have routed certain diseases, he also fires salvos at the drugs, technology, and amazing interventions of modern health care.

The crucial factors, he says, have involved advances in sanitation, and the environment remains the "primary determinant" of the health of any population.

He points, for instance, to the old childhood killers—scarlet fever, diphtheria, whooping cough, and measles. Almost 90 percent of the decline in death rates between 1860 and 1965 "occurred *before* the introduction of antibiotics and widespread immunization," he writes. "In part this recession may be attributed to improved housing and to a decrease in the virulence of microorganisms, but by far the most important factor was a higher host-resistance due to better nutrition."

"Host-resistance." That means the pathogens couldn't gain a toehold. It means the body is designed to vanquish or coexist with them. It means we can perform wondrous tasks without wonder drugs.

How?

That's the question Illich encouraged us to keep asking.

Two decades after Illich, Dr. Andrew Weil wrote his way onto the best-seller lists by making many of the same points. He cites studies that show conventional medicine is useful in only about 15 to 20 percent of cases. He reminds physicians-in-training, "You are not putting the cure back into a person. You are removing the obstacles to healing."[2]

Dr. Robert O. Becker, an orthopedist who has documented an "electromagnetic healing force," says, "The healer's job has always been to release something not understood, to remove obstructions (demons, germs, despair) between the sick patient and the force of life driving obscurely toward wholeness."[3]

---

1. From *Medical Nemesis: The Expropriation of Health* by Ivan Illich (New York: Pantheon Books, 1976), p. 15. Copyright © 1976 by Random House, Inc. Used by permission.
2. As cited in *Discovering the Body's Wisdom* by Mirka Knaster (New York: Bantam Books, 1996), p. 278. Copyright © 1996 by Mirka Knaster.
3. From "Weil: Life Medicine's Contrarian Crusader," in *Southwest Airlines Spirit* (January 1998): 44.

Daddy, the doctor I know best, likes to quote "the wise Frenchman" (whoever he is): "I only clean the wound. God does the healing."

On April 1, 1997, I found myself in a tiny examining room at Christ Hospital, waiting for a procedure to take me out of misery. Those blood clots in the vein under my collarbone had sprawled into other veins, despite a month of intense anticoagulant therapy. My right arm was bloated and red again, fingers stiff.

But it was my head that was doing me in. Florets of pain raked the creases of my brain. Narcotics only numbed the time between the flashes. I recalled childbirth; it seemed like a cakewalk.

Ann, a massage therapist, had come to our home the night before to give me a Reiki treatment. Her large hands moved slowly, meditatively, about six inches over me, attempting to normalize circulation and relieve pressure. I heard a crackling sound. The air seemed charged.

Never, I told myself, should I doubt that the body is an energy system or that matter is a configuration of energy. I tried to see electrons and protons spinning in the air above me. What am I—an accumulation of agreements between differing impulses?

As Ann worked, the pain softened and I relaxed deeply, yet I became surer about the dissonance in my brain. "Something is very wrong with me," I told her at the end, as I struggled to sit up.

Now, at the hospital, I was in a holding pattern. A CT scan of my brain revealed no bleeding or cancer. As soon as my oncologist finished with his other patients, I would go back to his office for removal of the Port-a-cath. Perhaps that would end my immune system's war on plastic. But first I needed fresh frozen plasma to reverse the effect of the blood thinners. Without it, I could bleed to death when he sliced open my arm.

Okay. What's another IV? I paid little attention to the nurses with their needles and bags of plasma. Yet as I sat there passively, telling myself "I can do this," I began to itch. First it was my stomach, then my back and legs, arms and neck. I pulled up my shirt. My skin was flaming red and covered with bumps.

My immune system had sniffed out another invader. I felt beleaguered by complications. I wasn't thinking about the cost, in dollars or cells, of another treatment-induced ailment. That realization came a couple of months later, when I looked in my folder of insurance company transactions and saw that more had been paid to correct the mistakes of treatment than on the treatment itself.

On that April Fool's Day I was just so weary. Yet in a bathroom mirror, I could still stare at my torso in awe.

Was this rash an example of what the Listener had said months earlier, "The immune system will follow the quality of intactness of the sense of self. Immune cells and nerve cells are so much the same. What's in the nervous system will be reflected in the immune system. They are never out of touch."

But could they communicate and act that quickly? The rash had appeared in no time.

Could I also heal with such speed? What would it take to restore my sense of self?

Dr. George Uetz is a biologist and a world authority on spiders. But when I went to interview him a few years ago at the University of Cincinnati, I was quite taken with his fly and beetle collection. I remember sitting in his office when he handed me a glass case full of dead insects, neatly arrayed and labeled. Offal eaters, I thought.

As if reading my mind, he said we rarely credit them for the service they perform in ridding the world of unneeded matter.

He learned that as a graduate student when he was hired to pick up road kills, put the deceased animals in cages, and document the insects that came to feed. What he discovered was not just a swarm of house-flies, as most people might suspect, but a distinct succession of insects, each performing a vital task.

A few years later he got a call from an investigator in the Hamilton County coroner's office. The guy was working a murder case and having difficulty determining the time of death. He wondered if Uetz could help by looking at the bugs on the corpse.

No problem. Uetz knew which insect should follow another, and could place the death within a critical forty-eight hours. Word of this circulated through the forensic community, and his phone began to ring more frequently. One day he got a call from a coroner in Indiana, who was working on a ritualized killing. The victim had been dismembered, and pieces of the body were disposed of separately, many miles apart.

That was the hypothesis, anyway. Investigators had to prove it.

But again, it was really no problem. Uetz could point to the same succession of insects, appearing at the same time on each limb. The beetles, in a sense, put the body back together.

I asked Uetz how this could be.

"They have spectacular nervous systems to detect the scent produced by decay."

March 12, 1998

> On the front page of the newspaper today is a story about pheromones—the chemical signals we exchange without realizing it. Scientists have known for decades that the menstrual cycles of women who live together often become synchronous. They don't need a couple of cycles to get in rhythm; they just sort of pull and push at each other's hormones until the rich blood appears.
>
> Now scientists are pinning this action to a substance in sweat. From armpit to nose to brain—is that how it goes? They can't say.
>
> So what, I ask, accounts for night sweats? Women going through menopause have been told that hot flashes and night sweats are caused by a surge of a hormone churned out by the pituitary gland. Sounds reasonable until you hear that women whose pituitary glands have been removed still get hot flashes.
>
> I like this line from the American Medical Association's book called *Women Health*: "Clearly, the underlying cause is not fully understood."[4]
>
> Perhaps it's something released from another woman's armpit and endured in tandem. Perhaps we, too, have spectacular nervous systems. We detect the scent of inadequacy, the decay of dreams. In sympathy, we burn.

---

4. From *Women's Health*, edited by Charles B. Clayman (Pleasantville, NY: The Reader's Digest Association, Inc., 1992), p. 152.

I like the story Dr. Oliver Sacks tells about the medical student in his book, *The Man Who Mistook His Wife for a Hat*. The young man swallowed a brew of recreational drugs, mostly amphetamines, which had an unexpected effect. He fell asleep, dreamed he was a dog, then woke to discover he had the olfactory system of one.

For the next three weeks he followed the impulses of his nose. "Infinitely redolent," he said, describing the world around him. He extolled the "happy smell of water . . . the brave smell of stone."[5] What he inhaled about a place or a person contained information as useful as what he gained by the use of his other senses.

Odors and scents fascinated him, then gradually overwhelmed and exhausted him. When the drug wore off, he felt relief, but also regret.

I used to think one of the worst diseases a person could have is insulin-dependent diabetes. All that attention to eating. All those needles. But when I had to give myself injections of anticoagulants twice daily, I learned what to do with sharpened steel, and I unlearned fear of diabetes.

"I am butter," I said to myself, looking at the place on my upper thigh or belly where I wanted to insert the needle. The loaded syringe rested on the surface of my skin. "I am butter. I am butter."

I waited, and somehow I would know when to exert the gentlest of pressure. The skin seemed to part. The syringe sank in. There was no pain and, later, no bruising.

I like what I can't explain—physicians who diagnose by the pulse, physicians who diagnose by the breath.

I like the fact that humans yawn when bored or tired, but never when angry, even if fatigue underlies their anger. I like goose bumps, which are a vestigial response of muscles that have not been needed for thousands of years.

I like me, with my left breast gone, no longer chilling on that side in a sharp wind. Men rub a woman's nipple as if it were a tiny penis; in fact it's more like a scrotum, protecting the juice within from the cold.

---

5. Reprinted with permission of Simon & Schuster, Inc., from *The Man Who Mistook His Wife for a Hat* by Oliver Sacks, p. 156. Copyright © 1970, 1981, 1983, 1984, 1985 by Oliver Sacks.

I like these words of Charles Darwin, quoted by Henry David Thoreau, "I took in February, three tablespoonsful of mud from three different points, beneath water, on the edge of a little pond; this mud when dried, weighed only [6.75] ounces. I kept it covered up in my study for six months, pulling up and counting each plant as it grew; the plants were of many kinds and were altogether 537 in number; and yet the viscid mud was all contained in a breakfast cup."[6]

I like the devotion of Luke Chan, a teacher of Chi Lel, a healing version of Tai Chi. When I visited him in his small office in suburban Cincinnati, he told me about a reunion he attended in Beijing with 150 people whose advanced cancer had been vanquished five years ago—"just doing Chi Lel." The slow, meditative movement he teaches "is not exhausting," he said. "It's nourishing. . . . But it must be continuous, like playing music. You never stop, because you love to do it." On very special days he does it for eight hours—without stopping.

I like what the guy told me who came to measure our driveway for fresh asphalt. "Isn't it amazing," I said, "the way weeds keep poking through the cracks?"

He nodded. "But not only the cracks," he said. "I saw a mushroom come up through six inches of asphalt. I don't know what it was about all that weight and heat that made it germinate. Do you know how hot it is when we lay that stuff down? About 275 degrees. I can't believe anything can stand that much heat."

Such things revive me in these days of certainty, when authorities are a dime a dozen, especially on talk radio, and known causes get leashed to demonstrable effects. The rest, seemingly, does not exist.

I especially liked meeting Kelly-Ann, a woman functioning with fragments of fifty-two personalities. Illnesses experienced, verified, and treated for one personality are not experienced, and hence need no treatment when another personality is holding sway.

That's why Kelly-Ann has a drawer full of glasses with different prescriptions and a closet jammed with clothes of clashing tastes. It's

---

6. Granted with permission from *Faith in a Seed: The Dispersion of Seeds and Other Late Natural History Writings*, Henry D. Thoreau, pp. 15–16. Copyright © 1993 by Island Press. Published by Island Press and Shearwater Books, Washington, DC and Covelo, CA. Used by permission.

not just her disposition and voice that change, but her pulse, blood pressure, blood chemistry, muscles, and organs.

The Listener says such people are great living treasures. They have so much to teach us about what we don't know: the way a personality can pull in weaknesses and strengths as if it were a magnet; the fluidity of matter, the healing potential of a new thought.

Kelly-Ann looked astonished and pleased when I told her this. She has been drugged, misdiagnosed, and hospitalized more times than she can remember. She has fought off labels of "crazy" and "disabled" that have shadowed her most of her adult life. She has tried several times to end her life.

No doctor has ever treated her like a treasure.

Lessons

April 4, 1997

Redbud blooming—It's a really lovely day. The sun
is pouring in, over my right shoulder, so warm and
comforting. I like this.

I like this: In the café at Joseph-Beth with Anne: cups
lined up on a tray behind the bar, under the coffee urns
and cappuccino machine. Matching, clean, they clink
when jostled.

I like the industry, intent, and knowledge behind
them. Coffee is good. Tea is good. How to serve it.

The light in the eye of our waitress.

The decades—no, centuries—of growers, processors.
Brown, rough burlap bags that hold beans. Places that
roast them.

The desire. The taste. The pleasure.

It is becoming clearer to me every day: We live
surrounded by miracles.

I wrote those words after surviving the clots, when the head pain
began to dissolve.

It is always easier to feel the extraordinary in the ordinary after side-
stepping death. I remembered leaving the hospital two days after the
mystery seizure.

October 18, 1996

It was late afternoon, blazing with color. Leaves halfway on, halfway
off. Air nippy. I couldn't imagine six months without driving, so I didn't
even try. I got on my bicycle, leaving my helmet in the garage, and
pumped as hard as I could around our village.

I pulled in the air and pushed it out with a yelp. Faster and harder,
faster and harder, giving into madness. Out of my way, you naysayers.

I still have life!

Seven weeks later, when the broken tubing was retrieved and people kept telling me how lucky I was to have survived five days with a foreign object in my heart, I had to find a pen. *(It is with shaky and grateful hands I write this date: December 5, 1996. "What a long strange trip it's been"— as the Grateful Dead would say. But I'm alive, into a new life. A nurse told me this was a "medical miracle." I believe it. She says it shows my heart muscle was very strong. Now I will run further and harder and sing when I walk.)*

Sometimes, when in the hospital or in the woolly stupor of chemo, I longed for the ordinary more than I ever have. I tried to settle the accounts of my life.

March 2, 1997

I want to run up the hood of a car, leap onto its roof, and raise my fists to heaven.

I want to become a ball in motion, not just the waiting mitt.

I want to blow through the trees, whip against your houses, whistle through the windows.

I want to be the letter that travels the globe to hands shaky with anticipation, a heart ravenous for words.

I want to build something stuck in the earth that lifts you into the sky.

I want to be welcome—as the aroma of coffee, the juice of an orange, the smooth comfort of chocolate.

I want to be more than I've been, more than I am, more than I've dared dream.

To feel better after feeling bad, to feel more whole while in pieces, to waken and sense all the promise of an unlived day: This is pretty intoxicating stuff. A woman who facilitates cancer support groups told me she likes being around people with life-threatening diseases. "I want what they've got," she said.

I nodded. She wasn't talking about cancer. She meant the altered mental state, the honeymoon infatuation with embodiment.

You take less for granted.
You take less s—.

You take less.
You take.
You give.
You give more.
You give more completely.
You give more for the heck of it.

This is sweet. But this is the baby food of personal change. The full feast is much richer, more textured, sometimes as bitter as a Moroccan olive.

I have no trouble waking up and feeling grateful. I'm a morning person and the daughter of a woman who counted her blessings daily, usually out loud over grapefruit sections and whole-wheat toast.

If she could not find something to affirm about someone, she invented reasons. She was always striking up conversations with strangers, telling the guy who washed our windows at a gas station in Michigan that he had a marvelous work ethic. ("Oh, please, Mother, not again, not here.")

I like the silence before dawn. I like its energy. I like to run around in my piece of the world and feel as if I own it. Then I like to come back, put on my clothes, and get to work.

The silence and deep darkness after midnight are difficult. The thoughts that bubble up, grab me, and sneer at sleep: These are more difficult. So, too, is the weight of my own heart, my uncertainty about forgiveness—how to do it, whether it happens. *(January 20, 1997: I can't let go. Another fear watches—that I will die sooner than I can open my heart, that the sum total of my life will be missed opportunities.)*

March 16, 1998

Looking back through the file labeled "Sessions with the Listener," I see that on February 7, 1997, he told our group: "The body is made for integration. In the natural movement toward it, there will naturally be impediments—blocks. But we can bring attention to those areas of blockage and discrepancy. This allows our own fluency to reestablish itself.

"The first and foremost thing is the attention. We must be gentle, compassionate and kind to ourselves. This can be actively fostered, as with a child or friend who really needs to be understood or accepted, but feels awkwardness or shame. And you, you could be there—respectful."

I can't believe he said it so long ago. I heard him, I thought, express this concept of self-acceptance ("If it were a child, you would not turn it away") just two months ago. But maybe that was the first time I heard it while in tune with what seems unacceptable in me.

I could touch that excruciating place with my mind. I could speak its peculiar logic with wonder, not cover my ears.

Early on during the group sessions I realized I'd never heard anyone talk as he does. Perhaps I've read ideas similar to his in a book, but not coming out of somebody's mouth—with ease, yet also conviction. That's why I took notes.

But notes are not enough. The timing has to be right. I will remain unconscious as long as I can.

I believe the adage: "When the student is ready, the teacher will come." But I also believe teachers are already here. Words written, but forgotten, in the margins of books. Something confessed by a close friend. Implied in the gesture of a spouse.

The teacher may be the fight two people always have. Not the content, but the form. The teacher may be a recurrent dream. The teacher may be a disease that can't be ignored. The teachers may be people who are dropped into our lives, to grope and growl and cheer with us—something we would not have done alone.

I am learning that a teacher lives within me. Someday I will stop ranting at God for supplying us with children without instruction books attached to them, or for supplying me with life without direction.

I will believe more in my sense and my love—common and accessible.

But I will always need the teachers who live outside me, nudging me on, suggesting books and tapes, sharing discoveries, offering a shift in perspective. In the aftermath of cancer, I needed the teachers who could make me unafraid of the path through darkness, unashamed of the times I drop to my knees, willing to talk and listen.

March 2, 1997

I have been blocked in trying to be brave, in thinking I had to detach. What I actually needed to do was attach, acknowledge that I'm feeling cruddy. Cry.

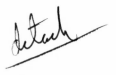

March 22, 1997

Blocks are funny things—physical or emotional or
spiritual. When they are in place and consciousness lies
on the downstream side of the block, then the mind—
receiving no water—begins to imagine the river never
existed. It's only after the block begins to be dissolved
and water starts to flow again that the memory of the river
returns and the effect of the block can be understood.

On March 2, 1998, my friend Emily loaned me a book she likes,
Tuesdays with Morrie. I did not read it. Still I did not read it. I finally
read it. Morrie, dying, talks to his old student, Mitch Albom. He tells
him he is detaching:

"Detaching yourself?"

"Yes. Detaching myself. And this is important—not just for someone like me, who is dying, but for someone like you, who is perfectly
healthy. Learn to detach."

He opened his eyes. He exhaled. "You know what the Buddhists say?
Don't cling to things, because everything is impermanent."

But wait, I said. Aren't you always talking about experiencing life?
All the good emotions, all the bad ones?

"Yes."

Well, how can you do that if you're detached?

"Ah. You're thinking, Mitch. But detachment doesn't mean you don't
let the experience *penetrate* you. On the contrary, you let it penetrate
you *fully.* That's how you are able to leave it."

I'm lost.

"Take any emotion—love for a woman, or grief for a loved one, or
what I'm going through, fear and pain from a deadly illness. If you hold
back on the emotions—if you don't allow yourself to go all the way
through them—you can never get to being detached, you're too busy
being afraid. You're afraid of the pain, you're afraid of the grief. You're
afraid of the vulnerability that loving entails.

"But by throwing yourself into these emotions, by allowing yourself
to dive in, all the way, over your head even, you experience them fully

51

and completely. You know what pain is. You know what love is. You know what grief is. And only then can you say, 'All right. I have experienced that emotion. Now I need to detach from that emotion for a moment.' "

Morrie stopped and looked me over, perhaps to make sure I was getting this right.

"I know you think this is just about dying," he said, "but it's like I keep telling you. When you learn how to die, you learn how to live."[1]

---

1. From *Tuesdays with Morrie: An Old Man, a Young Man, and Life's Greatest Lesson* by Mitch Albom (New York: Doubleday, 1997), pp. 103–104.

Gardening

In those group sessions, the women and I swapped tales. There was a juicy mix of black humor and indignation. As for empathy, the emotional state that purportedly fosters healing, I felt it from the beginning.

We shared oranges, chocolates from the women's separate travels, and often pastries. One of them couldn't seem to let a Halloween or St. Patrick's Day go by without sugar cookies, lavishly iced in the appropriate color.

We burned beeswax candles. We never sat in the same seat two sessions in a row. On very cold days, one of them brought hot water in a large thermos for tea. I would glance at my watch, not because I wanted our two hours to be over, only to savor the minutes.

None of our rituals and none of our sessions were planned. They just happened. At times, the unpredictability made me antsy.

We talked about cleansing cancer treatment of its own poisons. It wasn't an academic concern. It came out of anguish over life-threatening complications, disappointing surgeries, and the burden of fatigue, which increased with every hit of chemo.

The Listener listened.

Most people don't know that chemotherapy had its beginnings in the munitions industry of World War I. Germany had developed mustard gas, a compound that smells like mustard (though it has none in it), which can blister the skin, damage the lungs, and cause blindness or death. It also inhibits the production of white blood cells.

Someone figured out that this might be useful in the treatment of leukemia, which involves a proliferation of abnormal white blood cells. By the mid-fifties, the U.S. government put three million dollars into chemotherapy research, and a new kind of warfare was born.

Now systemic therapy is so standard and widespread, it's difficult to imagine cancer treatment without it. My oncologist, a fine, sincere man, would say that's good. "Only chemicals can kill cancer," he told me. He may be right—fully or partly. I don't know.

But undergo the treatment and the body screams foul. Women have had breast cancer for centuries. Surely some recovered without this, I whispered to myself in renegade moments. Those moments increased.

Once, I was disheartened after a tumor marker went up. I didn't know that one high result isn't particularly meaningful; it takes a series to set off alarms. All I knew was I had to get through a month before my blood could be retested. And that didn't feel good.

In an effort to comfort, a couple of acquaintances said, "Oh, you're going to be fine." I would nod in agreement as their hands seemed to wave me off.

But when a close friend said it too, I snapped. "You don't know that. I don't know that. But you want me to agree to what you are pretending to know so we can stop feeling bad about it."

My friend looked stunned.

As it turned out, I was fine.

But I didn't regret my words. Cancer patients have enough to carry. They don't need to shoulder somebody else's ungrounded optimism.

"Positive thinking"—the activity everybody says you must engage in if you want to get well—is a nosegay at best, a noose at worst.

A better response to a difficult development? A hug. Or, "I'm sure that's hard." Or, "I'm on your side."

True friends probably need no coaching. If their words don't say it, their actions do: "Whatever happens, I'm with you, every step of the way."

That is the balm in Gilead.

I told the group about going back for my first mammogram at the end of treatment. The last two times I'd been to the breast center, in the springs of 1993 and 1996, I'd had two breasts. Each time the center had issued me the all-clear. I was so thrilled I'd almost torn the letters to confetti. Such is the fear of breast cancer.

But my tumor, according to my surgeon, had been growing for eight years or more when I finally insisted that the hardness in my left breast wasn't normal.

So much for early detection. Something is wrong with this picture of mammography.

At the center I told myself to be polite, but forceful. My hand was shaking as I signed in at the front desk.

They were dealing with somebody to whom they'd given a false negative. I wasn't going to sue, but I wanted the technician to look in my eyes, look at my scars, and lopsided chest. I'm comfortable with my body, but each day I do a double take when I see just one breast in the mirror.

The technician seemed to find every place to look in the room except at me. Even when she was squeezing my right breast between the metal plates, she managed to use her fingers, not her eyes.

"We told you, you have dense breast tissue," she said, as if scolding me for a schoolyard infraction. "In women with dense breasts, malignancies are difficult to detect."

Actually, they had told me neither. I have the letter that proves it. But I was confused that day. I couldn't remember.

"Yes, you told me the first," I said to her. "But not the second. I learned that from my oncologist. He said it's like finding a snowball in a blizzard. But you guys never indicated any cause for concern. The letters said I had no irregularities. That's what I held onto."

She said she would instruct the radiologist to take extra care in the reading of my mammogram. She'd make sure he did it soon and understood my history. Yada yada yada.

I wasn't blaming her, but my heart was holding out for the two words that change everything: "I'm sorry."

They never came.

When our stories ended, The Listener would ask questions such as, "What serves your own intactness?" and "What do your bodies crave?"

The questions seemed almost subversive.

I was raised to distrust cravings. They get you into trouble. I mean isn't that why we pray, ". . . and lead us not into temptation"?

The Listener said the body knows what it needs. It is made for sufficiency; its systems want to be integral. He expressed his belief that we could tune into our cancer and what he called "the discrepancies" underlying it.

This allows our immune systems to become better acquainted with it. Then it better responds, adjusts, rectifies.

We could grow stronger around the tender place. Convalesce.

He encouraged us to meditate and taught simple techniques. He talked of the value of cultivating intuition and described the difference between being motivated by intuition and by a compulsion.

"Intuition comes in through a gateway of gentleness, though it may hit like a ton of bricks. With compulsion, there's a hardness, an agitation. Intuition stirs us, but there's not the same quality of agitation. Something comes together in a new way."

I realized that feeling good was good for my health.

The insight was absurdly modest. Yet it did bear its ton of bricks.

Again and again.

I didn't have to use my treatment or my fatigue as an excuse for not doing something I didn't really want to do. All I'd have to say was "no thanks."

I didn't need to have an idea seconded by someone else before I decided whether it was worth anything. All I'd have to say was, "I see it this way."

But I would have to live with myself for not pleasing someone, not seeking approval reflected back, not caring so much about judgment or rejection. This demanded change that reconfigured my DNA.

I have never described myself as a cripple. Why would I? I have two, perfectly functional legs that I enjoy using. Yet I was not carrying myself. I was living as a dependent on other people, putting their authority, respect, and affection ahead of my own.

I would have to nourish authentic self-love.

Someday, I would have to revisit the Lord's Prayer and those troublesome words I always shrank from, "lead us not into temptation." I would speak them again with comfort and conviction, "let me not be tempted to sell out on myself."

I began to reclaim my own authority in the group by closing my eyes or covering them when I talked. I couldn't explain why I was doing it. Like many of my actions, I don't understand them until later.

I made lists of things I enjoy and gave myself permission to do them, eat them, buy them, speak them. I tried to let intuition ripen, and I plucked its fruit. I kept discovering that when pain doesn't go away, it's time to sit with its agitation and listen for the shy message behind its noisy show.

Mostly, I relearned what I have always known. I crave silence. I like to be alone in our busy home when it isn't busy, when I can hear the creak of the pie safe in the living room and speak words as they come looking for a page.

Twenty years ago, I read Anne Morrow Lindbergh's *Gift from the Sea* for the first time. When a former colleague sent me a copy after my cancer was diagnosed, I put the book on a shelf. Now I reopen it and feel understood:

> If one sets aside time for a business appointment, a trip to the hairdresser, a social engagement, or a shopping expedition, that time is accepted as inviolable. But if one says: I cannot come because that is my hour to be alone, one is considered rude, egotistical, or strange. What a commentary on our civilization, when being alone is considered suspect; when one has to apologize for it, make excuses, hide the fact that one practices—like a secret vice![1]

The Great Physician said:

> "Listen! A sower went out to sow. And as he sowed, some seed fell on the path, and the birds came and ate it up. Other seed fell on rocky ground, where it did not have much soil, and it sprang up quickly, since it had no depth of soil. And when the sun rose, it was scorched; and since it had no root, it withered away. Other seed fell among thorns, and the thorns grew up and choked it, and it yielded no grain. Other seed fell into good soil and brought forth grain, growing up and increasing and yielding thirty and sixty and a hundredfold." (Mark 4:3–8)

The Listener asked us to design a treatment plan that would meet more of our needs than current therapies do. We said it should involve both group and individual psychotherapy, massage, Healing Touch,

---

1. From *Gift from the Sea* by Anne Morrow Lindbergh (New York: Pantheon Books, 1975), p. 44. Copyright © 1955, 1975 by Anne Morrow Lindbergh. Used by permission.

maybe acupuncture, nutrition counseling, and some education on the nature of disease, and the intelligence of the body.

He suggested a second tier of therapy for those who might want to do more intense inner work. He described a process of becoming attentive to the places where one is stuck. He used the example of anger, how rethinking what made us angry can revive the anger. But that's not enough.

If we can bring the attention of the mind to the place in the body where anger (or grief, guilt, or shame) is housed, then it's possible to feel the sensation release. We become unstuck.

"You can access the energy entrapped in the angry thought and use it for other things."

I fantasized about a facility where various services would be available, fanning out around a central courtyard like spokes in a wheel. Art classes, chi qong, massage, movement classes, chemotherapy, radiation therapy, a bookstore and juice bar, a butterfly garden for sitting and digging. No one modality would dominate, but each would have a respected function.

I wanted it to be splendid and inspiring, like a great school, retreat center, or mountain.

As we brainstormed, I realized it wouldn't need to be just for people with cancer or other serious diseases, or those close to the end.

The sick parts and the well parts of me could sing this part in harmony: It would be for anyone. It would be for life.

Nine months later, I interviewed Susan Love when she came to Cincinnati for an evening address sponsored by one of the hospital conglomerates and insurance company. She is a smart, gritty, passionate surgeon. But the quality I appreciate most is her candor. She lets you know where her facts and abilities end.

"We understand so little about breast cancer," she told me. "It's like the blind man and the elephant. We only know about one toenail."

She compared our knowledge of the many diseases categorized under the heading "breast cancer" to what our knowledge of tuberculosis was *before* the disease was linked to the organism *Mycobacterium tuberculosis*. She shuddered as she spoke.

She didn't try to gloss over the inadequacies of treatment. "Surgery, chemo, and radiation are crude ways to deal with a disease, let's face it.

But if I were diagnosed tomorrow, I'd sign up for every minute of slash, burn, and poison." That's to cover the bases, she explained.

She has seen both deaths and survivals that defy explanation. After twenty years of practice she refuses to make predictions anymore. Nevertheless, she predicted that the work of a researcher in San Francisco could revolutionize treatment.

The woman's discoveries were based on a simple exchange. She took cancer cells out of a diseased breast and placed them into healthy tissue.

"Guess what? They behaved benignly," said Dr. Love, beaming. "The future isn't going to be with a war mentality. Maybe it won't be in killing cancer, but controlling it or putting it to sleep for a long time. The secret may be to just change the environment and then rehabilitate the cells."

Managing

May 14, 1997

> Back at the hospital for more tests—x-ray, CT scan,
> MRI, and mammogram. Bones clean, I think. That's
> what the tech indicated.

EEG showed I still have that temporal lobe abnormality. Dilantin continues. Oh well. Worse things could be happening.

I was sitting in the radiation department waiting room. These tests, at the end of chemo, were going to tell me whether my cancer was stronger, more mischievous than the chemicals they'd been shooting into my veins for nine months.

I was not interested in the magazines stacked on the table beside me or in other people's conversations.

I usually like to eavesdrop. In every reporter lives a cowardly spy. One day two women, sitting behind me, heads tipped together, were chatting about the TV show *Ellen*. One of them, quite matter-of-factly said she was thinking of coming out at work.

The other yawned and just as matter-of-factly responded, "Fine, honey. I'm stopping at the dry cleaners on the way home. Got anything you want me to pick up?" I pinched myself. Since when has Cincinnati become so relaxed about sexual orientation?

But on this day my snooping gene was upstaged by my anxiety genes. I knew I needed to let them pull together and speak. My journal lay open across my lap.

> Without desiring it I have been plunged into that
> thought pool where the big what-ifs swim. What if they
> find more? What if I face death when the boys are
> young?
> After all these months of chemotherapy, I still have
> problems with it—conceptualizing its efficacy, getting
> over the barbarism implicit in any form of poisoning.

60

It's just a latter-day version of leeches, although that frankly seems more natural (sucking out diseased blood, thereby altering its ratios).

Here's my problem with current cancer therapy: It's retrospective.

It deals with already manifested events, tainted matter. Yet what oncologists know is that cancer is a dynamic disease, a potentiality that can remanifest itself. Surgery makes sense to me. You cut out a wad of haywire cells. Chemotherapy makes a kind of sense, too, if it's only going after the already created cells.

But what long-term chemotherapy operates on is the understanding that cancerous cells are going to continue to be created. So the chemo courses through the body, prepared to ambush the bad-boy cells when they hatch and try to reproduce. The only reason chemotherapy works and doesn't kill people outright is that the cancer cells are slightly weaker than other cells in the body.

Bone marrow transplants push this paradigm to the limit—harvest bone marrow, kill everything in sight, reintroduce bone marrow, and hope the patient can survive. I understand why a person in this state can fall prey to a variety of diseases, including more cancer.

Why?

Because the immune system has been sucker-punched.

Because the "underlying discrepancy," as The Listener calls it, which allowed the initial cancer to grow, has not been changed.

Therefore, it's a flawed procedure.

I'm not a scientist. I didn't take enough classes in high school or college even to speak the language. I remember when my oncologist described cancer as "a genetic disturbance," I felt disappointed. I wanted a grander sense of mystery.

It took me months to realize that the understanding I had groped my way toward empirically, that cancer is "a potentiality that can remanifest itself," was a clumsy way of saying "genetic disturbance."

I felt that the only time one could speak of "curing" cancer would be after testing a person's DNA to see if the mutation had corrected itself. But I know of no such test.

Physicians use the word *remission*, not *cure*, when they speak of the absence of detectable cancer. This seems honest to me. They are chasing troubled cells, not re-creating perfect ones. But most of us don't hear "remission" or, if we do, we think it means "cure."

The surveillance work of physicians is driven by numbers: A breast tumor, roughly one centimeter in diameter, is the product of nearly a decade of cell divisions. They know that by the time a tumor becomes palpable, cells probably have broken free, done the Australian crawl through the bloodstream, and may be clinging to a femur or hiding in a pocket of the brain.

They know the average replicating rate of these cells. They know that if enough replications occur, such that a tenth of the body's eleven trillion cells have turned cancerous, death is imminent.

So why don't they tell people the truth? "You have a chronic disease."

Or, "You probably have a chronic disease." *Probably* leaves room for actual cures, which we know even less about than partial ones.

Chronic diseases are managed and lived with—sometimes quite well. But my longtime friend with multiple sclerosis and my new friend with diabetes must be active with themselves each day. They are not waiting for a crisis before taking care of themselves.

I tell Amy, whose multiple sclerosis was diagnosed when she was sixteen and still dreaming of a career on a stage, that if I lived at her pace I would be dead in a month. She's an attorney who adores the arts and supports local artists by going to the ballet and theater, concerts, lectures, and gallery openings, often five nights a week.

Talk drains me; it energizes her. To me it is chit-chat. To her it is a means to lasting connections.

I suspect she looks at the hours I keep and the solitude I need and groans. She would feel punished to live my life.

Are certain lifestyles better, morally or physiologically, than others?

I used to think so, when I nibbled my bran muffins, went on my daily runs, and felt none of the compulsions that sweep other people into passion plays. Then I felt the power of my own compulsions, and I realized I need to leave such questions to doctors or theologians.

I need to shrug more often when I see someone with a doughnut in one hand, a cigarette in the other, and a pristine bill of health. I need to concern myself less with absolute truths and more with my own.

What works for me? What fits?

A few days after the testing, I went back to the group, still uncertain about what the MRI and other exams had revealed. But I knew what I felt, and what I felt was no more chemo. If the cancer was going nuts, partying in my organs, chewing my bones, I still wanted to try something different.

Would they support me? I had asked the same of Paul and other close friends.

The women smiled and nodded. The Listener too. Even his office, with its hearth, its chevron windows of leaded glass, his array of arcane trinkets, seemed to welcome my odd request in a familiar way. I guess I had known that it wouldn't matter if they thought I was crazy.

They would not abandon me. Nor would they try to argue me into the corner labeled self-doubt.

As I was leaving, I asked The Listener if I could make an appointment for some individual therapy. For nine months I'd followed conventional medical wisdom. I'd done somebody else's treatment, accepted all their needles and swallowed all their pills.

Now I wanted to design a strategy for optimal health and guide it myself.

I was ready to get prospective about cancer.

It was then that my little pot began to boil, that the word *porridge* rose in me, and I discovered that the tools of my livelihood and the wanderings in my journal are the very marrow of my life.

September 17, 1997

> Circle game:
> I hurt.
> Therefore I write.
> I write.
> Therefore I don't hurt.
> I don't hurt. I don't write.
> I don't write. I hurt.
> Therefore . . .

Some people see jewels in rain. In water they are reborn. Some people can stroke the petal of a rose in only a handful of clay. In dirt they create. Some people feel the tensile strength in a chord and weave rifts. Paul is one of them.

Words birth me and lead me. I reach for them and hold them as if they were runes.

And yet, eleven months after that, when the group ended and my heart felt like a balloon flying adrift, it was this image that kept me going: I am falling back into space. No one stands behind me. My fingers loosen on my pages. They blow into the wind and the words fly off.

Now that is courage. That too is a way Home.

But I am scared of that way.

Letting Go

On December 10, 1997, I went to Dr. Mary Glass's chiropractic office as a reporter. This means she was talking and I was listening, filling up pages in my skinny notebook. I was there because a therapist I know said Dr. Glass does some amazing things based on "contact reflex analysis," which she refers to as CRA. It's a way of collecting data from a body's reflex points.

What are reflex points?

The information sheet she gave me explained that they're "derived from the ancient Chinese system of acupuncture. . . . It is a study of how the different points on the surface of the body relate to the state of health and the flow of energy in each and every function and part of the body."

If a CRA practitioner touches a "hot" reflex point, she said, then energy is transferred from that spot to the test muscle on an arm, making it weaken and drop. That's the clue to an imbalance of some sort.

Perhaps she saw a look of uncertainty pass over my face because she acknowledged that it would be difficult to understand her analytical technique, if I didn't see her interact with a patient.

I nodded. Even her examining room was a challenge for me. Where was the sink? The lemony-scrubbed smell? The scales and little privacy curtain? The meds locked behind glass? I was measuring it against my memories of the office where my father, an internist, was the king dressed in a starched lab coat.

My brother-in-law, Bruce, who died at forty-three in a plane crash, was a chiropractor. He was at ease touching people. He gave great hugs and his broad fingers had confidently adjusted my neck many times. But I'd never been in his office, never experienced how a chiropractor works.

I know my father must have swallowed hard when my sister started dating a chiropractor. Medical doctors and chiropractors, in the era of my youth, were like Capulets and Montagues. We did not mix. My parents, following the medical doctor's company line, viewed them as unhealthy competitors at best, quacks and knaves at worst. When one Oriental chiropractor had the nerve to advertise in our weekly newspaper, we kids put on phony accents and raved about curing cancer. We played for laughs at Dr. Wong's expense.

But Bruce won over Daddy. Maybe because he didn't try. My father's view toward chiropractors softened; he allowed that they could be useful with certain back problems. He was pleased when his orthopedic colleagues made referrals. But dissolve kidney stones? Reverse heart disease? Shrink a tumor?

I'm scared to ask. I think his eyes would still roll.

Dr. Glass's office contains various charts of the body, viewing it as a skeletal system, a muscular system, and a network of nerves, vessels, and organs. She also has a life-size model of the spine, a bookcase in one corner, a desk in the other. The centerpiece of the room is her adjustment table. The space feels scholarly; it's neat and clean, but not antiseptic.

It was lunch hour and there were no patients in the lobby. "Would you want me to show you what I do?"

"On me?"

"Yes, you. You're having some discomfort right here, aren't you?" she said, laying her hand gently upon the middle of my back.

I was stunned. When I woke up that morning I'd felt fine, but about an hour before our appointment the muscles in the middle of my back began to ache. It was a familiar sensation, something that would come and go. I remembered a nightmare: A stranger tries to touch that place in my back. If he touches it hard enough, I will die. He gets me in his grasp. I twitch. He increases the pressure. I begin to gasp and scream. I wake up.

The stranger's face changes. But the dream returns, year after year. I realize I'd had the dream again, just the week before. Now I felt the ache. Maybe if she gave me an adjustment, pushed hard and something cracked, well, maybe the ache and the dream would go away forever.

"Yes, sure, that would be fine," I said.

She asked me to sit, not lie, on the table and stick out my left arm, locking it at the elbow. Then she began lightly pressing and releasing places all over my body. I was sure her analysis would inspire her to do a snap-crackle-pop on my spine. But she said my body was telling her it wanted to release a memory.

My body telling her? Release a memory? This was an unfamiliar language. But I was game. Reporters have to be.

She had already told me that her practice began to change a few years ago after sitting down and identifying some dissatisfaction within herself. "With straight chiropractic I was getting some of the people well some of the time." By *straight chiropractic* she meant biomechanical manipulation, primarily of the spine.

She wanted to better the percentages. For one thing, she had to increase patient participation—results correspond to how well the patients follow the recommendations. But was there anything she could do to jump-start the process?

A former colleague told her about Contact Reflex Analysis and the system of nutritional support that goes with it. In 1995, she trained with the Michigan chiropractor who began developing CRA forty years ago. She was impressed, she said, by improvements in patients. "Then I began learning about the neuroemotional system and how powerful the mind is."

She learned a technique, pioneered by another doctor, to help subconscious thoughts enter into consciousness, and she blended these methods into her practice as well. Again, she said, results have been impressive.

"What I do is ask the body what is wrong," she said. "The body will talk to you before a situation becomes pathological. But most people don't listen. They don't know how."

In my case, Dr. Glass believed that "something within the body memory is taking energy from the conscious brain. We need to identify it. Do you want to?"

Sure. What did I have to lose? Sore muscles, I hoped.

She continued her analysis, touching and releasing points, around my face, back, and arms. Finally, she said, "This is about something that occurred when you were sixteen or seventeen, something you did that affected someone else. What might that be?"

I shrugged. Then a thought came without effort. "I got kicked out of boarding school."

"So?" she said, puzzled. "Did that affect someone else?"

Her question was like the beam of a flashlight illuminating a crawl space. "I disappointed my mother," I said, surprised and suddenly sorrowful. Tears filled my eyes. Dr. Glass left the room in search of a box of tissues.

I never cry in front of strangers, not even at the end of movies. I rub out the tears or pretend I'm really interested in the credits on the screen.

She returned. "Well, it's out now. Let it go."

I was shaking my head. That word that had come out of my mouth, *disappointed*, was new. I'd never seen the situation that way before. In every retelling of the events that led up to that headmaster's letter, requesting I not return to Westtown School, I spoke like an adolescent giddy with self-assurance.

What a repressive place. What a stupid decision.

My stories of the rules I broke, the punishment I endured, my secret friendship with a teacher had always been met with laughter from other people, or a shake of the index finger and mummerings of admiration. My antics may have impressed them, but I guess I'd never really convinced myself. These tears were showing me that.

I couldn't seem to laugh away the one woman whose heart had been broken by her daughter's rebellion.

Or had it? I will never know for sure. Perhaps that's why the tears felt barbed, opening a reluctant place in my heart.

I can never test my guilt against her forgiveness. My mother died when I was nineteen.

"Let it go," Dr. Glass repeated. "Let it go."

Lost and Found

I was lost.

No. Let me try that again: I thought I was lost. Maybe I was just stuck. I couldn't seem to move because I had forgotten where I was going and why I wanted to get there.

Even the ground under my feet seemed suspect. I had a dream of nearly dying, then coming home, walking in and not being wanted. The boys had taken all their toys into the yard, and kids I didn't even know were running in and out. Paul was sitting in a room playing music with strangers, smoking cigarettes. He glared at me.

Paul has never smoked.

Memories of feeling awkward in social settings paraded in front of me, thumbing their noses. I thought of going alone to a prom. Going alone to a wedding reception. Meeting the new boss who decided to take away my column. Nervous sweat rolled down the sides of my torso. I felt as if I was deep underwater, drowning.

"Life is a continual dance with change, impermanence, and loss," writes Christine Longaker, a Buddhist, a pioneer in the hospice movement and author of *Facing Death and Finding Hope*. "When we really look into our most painful life experiences, then, we realize that death is no stranger to us. Even though death may seem like a remote event that will be unlike anything we've experienced, we actually suffer many losses in the midst of life that feel as uncompromising as death itself."[1]

I remembered "the secret" my older brother and sister disclosed to me one night when I was young, probably four or five: "You were adopted. Left on our doorstep."

My parents were out for the evening and the sitter was in the kitchen, washing dishes. My eyes widened, stomach twisted. "I had to

---

1. From *Facing Death and Finding Hope* by Christine Longaker (New York: Doubleday, 1997), p. 47. Copyright © 1997 by Christine Longaker and Rigpa Fellowship.

get rid of my dog because of you," my brother reminded me. "I want my dog back."

I panicked for my parents to return—in the dark, sheet pulled up to my nose, listening for their car, waiting for a beam of light to turn into the driveway. Anne asleep in the bed next to mine.

My mother always paused at our door to hear our breathing before she entered. My voice stretched for her. "Was I adopted?"

"What?" She sat on my bed, parted my bangs and kissed me on the forehead. "Don't you remember? You were two weeks past the due date. It was so hot that summer, and I so big. I was miserable. Auntie Gretchen came on the train for your birth, but she couldn't wait that long. She left the day before. When you were born, you cried and cried."

"That's why you got rid of Bill's dog?"

"Read the Beatitudes," Dr. Mary Glass suggested.

After our interview I had decided to return as a patient. But I hadn't said anything about this anxiety of not belonging.

How could I? It simmered under the surface of conscious thought, more like an ache than a pain. Dr. Glass had identified it through reflex testing and by using her "neuroemotional" techniques.

"The Beatitudes?" I said. "The fifth chapter of Matthew?"

"Yes," she said. "Don't forget."

I thought I knew that long, paradoxical, "blessed are" passage by heart. But I couldn't understand why she would tell me to read it. So I read it again.

> Blessed are those who mourn, for they will be comforted.
> Blessed are the meek, for they will inherit the earth.
> Blessed are those who hunger and thirst for righteousness,
>   for they will be filled.
> Blessed are the merciful, for they will receive mercy.

Every one of those blessed souls has roots and belongs—not to places or to power, but to ways of being, to their own desires, to their grief and love, to God.

I realized then: What I am really looking for is a place where I will never feel like an outsider.

January 18, 1998

Home is where:
    the light glows yellow in the kitchen;
    the best blankets are the old, soft ones;
    there's always room at the table for another;
    silence is profound;
    privacy is prized like a jewel;
    things are always being made—words on a page,
      music, bread;
    many hands make light of spilled milk;
    "I'm sorry" is cause for celebration and "I will try" is
      encouraged with a hug;
        confusion, grief, and shame are welcome
        (because the worst shame is being ashamed of
        shame);
Home is where God can belch or pad about in
    stocking feet.
Home is where I live.
Home is not about mortgage payments, insurance,
    and taxes. It's about purpose, but it's not purpose.
Home is not shelter. It's what shelter allows us to do
    and be when we have it.

Two weeks later I returned to Dr. Glass's office. She asked me if I'd read the Beatitudes. "It wasn't really that passage that I wanted you to see, but the one that comes next," she said. "You know, the one about not hiding your light. It's a message to all of us."

The Physician says:

> You are the light of the world. A city built on a hill cannot be hid. No one after lighting a lamp puts it under the bushel basket, but on the lamp stand, and it gives light to all in the house. (Matt. 5:14–15)

Going Home

I might describe Paula's studio as dowdy, if I didn't know how much it means to her—or, if her paintings and prints did not cover the walls and circle the baseboards.

The wood floors are scuffed bare in places and splattered with paint. The exposed beams and light fixtures are functional. They make no architectural statements. The rambling, former factory in Northside that contains Paula's space looks like a good idea never pushed to completion.

Oh well. The lights work. The toilet down the hall flushes. Other artists come and go.

"I got the studio a year-and-a-half ago," Paula told me. "As I drove over here the first time, my car packed with supplies, I kept saying, 'I'm going home. I'm going home.' The words sounded so right."

And so odd, if you could see her sturdy, brick, high-ceilinged home, about five miles away, with bright-colored walls, her gorgeous paintings, a grand piano, a vintage car in the garage, gardens front and back.

But right, yes. Her studio is home.

We had been talking for nearly two hours when she said that, my mind growing dull by so much stimulation. But the words jerked me to attention. This was my issue. Where do I belong?

I searched out that kids' book by Mary Ann Hoberman, *A House Is a House for Me*, and was surprised to find the page I wanted dog-eared.

> A box is a house for a teabag,
> A teapot's a house for some tea.
> If you pour me a cup and I drink it all up,
> Then the teahouse will turn into me![1]

---

1. From *A House Is a House for Me* by Mary Ann Hoberman (New York: Puffin Books, 1987). Reprinted 1983 (twice), 1984 (twice), 1985, 1986, 1987.

It's what goes on inside a place that defines it. When these goings on feed, comfort, and inspirit, then the place is a home, not only for free expression but also healing.

"Only recently have I been able to say, 'I'm an artist.' I always felt art was on this higher plane," she said. "But now I think we all are artists—even before you pick up a paintbrush."

For most of her adult life she woke up in the morning, looked in the mirror and said, "I'm a physician." The title made her a bit skeptical of herself, even though she cherished being a part of patients' lives, hearing their stories, conducting their care.

Dr. Paula Fletcher, graduate of the University of Kentucky Medical School, was a family practice physician for nearly twenty years until she became so sick that she had to walk out of her Kenwood office one night, never to return.

The disease that nearly killed her was a rare blood disorder called primary amyloidosis. It was July 1990 when she noticed how tired she was during the day and how many times she wakened at night to urinate. Suspecting a couple of treatable ailments, perhaps a hyperactive thyroid, she ordered tests on her own blood and urine.

They revealed startling abnormalities, pointing to a disease so unusual she'd never encountered it in a patient before. For unknown reasons her plasma cells were going haywire, producing a protein that would cram into her liver and kidneys and not go away.

She tried to research the disorder, which is sometimes classified as a blood cancer, but all she could see were faces of patients with either kidney or liver disease. She knew how much they suffered.

"I sat on the floor of the bookstore and cried. I couldn't put it into my consciousness."

She consulted colleagues and a favorite medical school professor. They pointed her to the Mayo Clinic, one of two centers in the United States specializing in primary amyloidosis. But the inescapable reality was that people don't live with the disease.

A couple of months. Maybe a year or two. That's all she'd have.

I winced as Paula told me this. But she spoke with the detachment of a clinician. Her look did not mirror mine. Nor did she get swept into the drama of the disease—as some people do. It seems to be the low they get high on.

Her treatment consisted of a potion of medications aimed at stopping the faulty proteins from bedding down in her liver, kidneys, or other organs. The strict regimen kept her on the edge of intestinal distress. "I got worse and worse and they kept upping the dose. Then at Mayo they were talking about evaluating me for a liver transplant. I said, 'No, my platelets are too low for a biopsy.' But really, I just didn't want it. "I went home. Then I started getting better."

It wasn't dramatic. The turnaround took months. She continued chemotherapy until her bone marrow could tolerate no more. Formerly a vegetarian, she had returned to eating meat because she needed 130 grams of protein a day—more than triple the normal amount.

She found herself thanking the animals whose bodies were sustaining her body. At the same time, she thanked the once normal cells that were being destroyed and excreted. She knew they contained calcium, amino acids, essential elements.

Incapable of doing any good inside of her, they would return to the earth for recycling. "I was never comfortable with the idea, 'I'm sending this in to kill a part of my body.' Expressing thanks gave me some kind of resolution.

"I believe all cells have intelligence. So I spoke to my immune system. I said, 'I know this will be hard. I appreciate what you're doing. I want you to know I'm going to be silent and listen to what you need. But I'm not very practiced in this, so you may have to tell me again.' "

In one of those hushed dialogues the answer surprised her. It seemed almost silly. "Green. I need green." She answered by eating a green pepper every day, as well as broccoli and spinach and cabbage, and she couldn't resist painting the living room of her Hyde Park home green.

When the answer came "red," she painted the kitchen a deep coral. By the time yellow came, only a bathroom was left.

She laughs about these indulgences, but they paralleled significant other ones. Paula can't remember a time in her life when she didn't play piano or sketch on the edges of texts. It was natural that with some free time on her hands she would sign up for an art class.

But when the teacher came around after she put one line on her paper and said, "That's wrong," Paula stopped.

"My first response was, 'Start over.' My second response was, 'Do I really want to be here?' No. I didn't. I packed up my things and left. It was one of the most freeing things I've ever done."

Early on in her illness she'd made a pact with herself "to be as attentive as I could, not to run away from myself." The art class experience did not shut down her creativity.

It encouraged her defiance, hastened her development. She kept on sketching and painting and trying new media without worrying about a right or wrong way. Her studio and home are alive with her work, as well as the music and books that have nourished it.

"I've found parts of myself I didn't even know were there. It's more like what it was when I was a kid, growing up on a farm in central Kentucky—taking joy in little things, like the first buds in the spring." In her 1997 book *Living Color*, writer/painter Natalie Goldberg tells a story she loves—how Henri Matisse became an artist.

> A law clerk, he began painting at the age of twenty while he was convalescing from appendicitis at his parents' home. Little more than a year later, in 1890, he abandoned law altogether and went to Paris to study art. Painting, he said, opened for him "a kind of paradise" set apart from ordinary life. . . . He let himself be seduced by pleasure. It was his guide and he followed it. Pain is not the only way we can learn.[2]

For Paula, her weird disease opened a door for her that nothing else had. First, it forced her to acknowledge that she had not been taking care of herself. She let the demands of a busy practice shape each day, week, year.

With her life threatened, she had to take stock of the activities she liked and do them. Her time felt so limited. Gradually, she found her true center in art and music, translating ideas into form, color, and sound. In addition to her piano, she is learning banjo and singing in a women's chorus.

It's not that art is magical. It's that art led her to her inner oasis, a place of zest and harmony. That, she is convinced, is essential to healing.

---

2. From *Living Color* by Natalie Goldberg (New York: Bantam Books, 1997). Copyright © 1997 by Natalie Goldberg.

Paula spends her days in the studio or hiking through Spring Grove Cemetery, sketching statuaries. "I can't wait to get here and I can't stand to leave."

The best case scenario, offered to her in 1990, was twenty-four more months. She's had more than ninety months and the clock's still ticking. Why did she survive? Why, when her liver and kidney were drowning in deranged cells, did her body take a U-turn and slowly, obstinately drive toward health?

Was it two years of chemotherapy that saved her? the mega-protein diet? group sessions at the Wellness Community? the visualizations? the colors?

"One doc says it was chemo. Another says the chemo didn't do a thing for me. He said it was all the other stuff I was doing. I believe it was a combination."

Caryle Hirshberg and Marc Ian Barasch, authors of the 1995 book, *Remarkable Recovery*, argue that such cases are really not so rare and deserve scrutiny. "Certainly, some aspects of these people's bodies, minds, or even spirits must have accounted for the outcome,"[3] they write.

"But we cannot begin to know if we do not designate such instances as remarkable enough to warrant further study, if we do not crack a very exclusive club to include people who had previously fallen into a medical gray area."

Paula's health is stable, though she still has to be careful about fatigue and continues to monitor proteins in her urine, which reflect the activity of her blood.

What do her physicians say about how she has outlived their most generous predictions and found a richer life?

"They're amazed. I am too."

---

3. From *Remarkable Recovery: What Extraordinary Healings Tell Us about Getting Well and Staying Well* by Caryle Hirshberg and Marc Ian Barasch (New York: Riverhead Books, 1995), p. 18. Copyright © 1995 by Caryle Hirshberg and Marc Ian Barasch.

Foreign Bodies

I wish I could say that my back quit hurting after that first impromptu session with Dr. Glass. It actually ached for a few days.

But I felt lighter, freer. Almost giggly. And very curious.

What was going on with my back?

I'd always assumed that muscle pain is a result of overexertion, misuse, or poor posture. I believed that those nightmares came from a spasm of some sort. Some day I would remember to ask a doctor: Is there a trigger spot on the human back? Touch it and you die?

The spasm would be over by the time I woke up. That made it different from a charley horse, which yanks me out of sleep and tightens its grip as consciousness increases, or a stomach flu, which kicks my gut all the way to the toilet.

I had never given the back stuff much thought, nor comforted it with more than an occasional muscle relaxant. I probably just need more water, I'd tell myself.

This could be the only solution I will ever need. But I felt an urgency I'd never experienced before. Something in me wanted to be known.

The nightmare was sandwiched between other desperate dreams. Sometimes I'd get caught in a place between sleeping and waking. I could see myself lying on the bed. I could see someone coming up our stairs. I would call to Paul to wake up. Wake up! But nothing came out of my mouth.

Was this a memory? a metaphor? a meaningless phantasm of sleep?

The Adventurer wanted answers. The Skeptic snorted in disapproval. The skeptic was my father and every professor and almost every boss I have ever had.

The Adventurer won.

Suppose I approached my back as a scientist might. I could take note of the where and when of discomfort. I could close my eyes and let my attention go to it. I could describe it, draw pictures of it, converse with it.

What did I have to lose?

When Owen was eight and Noah five, we took them sledding behind Hal and Betty's house on New Year's Eve. After racing up and down the golf course hills, we went inside for snacks. There, under the influence of cocoa and the crackle of a fire, the boys began to whoop it up, sliding in stocking feet on the waxed wood floors.

On one run, Owen's sock caught a snag of wood. He went down, pulling up a twelve-inch dagger of oak that somehow speared him in the rump. Paul snatched the wood out of Owen's pants, but his screams and flailing hands made us realize he was impaled.

Children's Hospital gave us fast-track service that afternoon. A doctor made an inch-long slice in Owen's buttock and pulled out a splinter that went two inches deep. He then used just one suture to close it. "We want the wound to stay sort of open. That's in case there are other splinters we can't see," he explained.

Sure enough, several days later a few pieces floated to the surface, and we washed them away. The wound filled in strong and white, slightly mounded. We milked the incident for all the gasps we could get. Owen smiled shyly at each retelling.

Months went by. Nine, to be precise. Owen was in the upstairs bathroom whisking off his clothes for a bath before bed. Out of the corner of my eye I noticed that his white scar looked raised and red. I didn't say anything, but after he got finished in the bath, I asked Paul to inspect it.

Under the surface of the skin, Paul felt something hard. He squeezed and out popped the last chunk of oak, about a quarter-inch square. This time the wound healed flat and the white skin melted into pink.

I thought of Owen's butt when I went to work on my back.

December 12, 1997

> I'm not suffering, though my back is hurting. It's a funny kind of discomfort, emanating from a core, a knot.

Sometimes, lying still, I can get into it and let it fan out, filling the cavity of my chest and torso. The only way to peace is through greeting the pain, not shrinking from it, acquainting myself with it.

Several weeks later I decided to try a couple of sessions of Eye Movement Desensitization and Reprocessing (EMDR) therapy after I did a story about it for the paper. "Why are you here?" the counselor asked me.

"Because of my back," I said.

That wasn't the typical response. Most people would identify a trauma or an emotional issue they needed to work through. But the therapist adapted my physical symptom to the protocol. EMDR is a technique that stimulates the brain bilaterally to help it shake free of snags and blocks. It uses blinking lights, alternating tones, or the movement of a therapist's hands.

The alternating tones seemed best suited for me. When I put on a headset, focusing on the beep-beep, beep-beep and feeling the tension in my back, I traveled quickly to a place of terror and torture.

Spasms of I-don't-know-what uncurled in me. I twitched and gasped, much as I have in my dreams. She watched in astonishment and with some concern that I might be on the verge of a seizure.

She stopped the equipment. "See anything? Recognize anyone? Hear anything?"

"No." All I saw were colors, opening like flowers.

But, again, when I left I felt lighter, freer. "Like a nice housecleaning," I told her.

In the following days and weeks, I noticed that the back pain would come and go, with no relationship at all to exertion. A stressful situation could bring it on, while a minute or so of gentle attention could take it away. I lived under the embrace of hot rice packs.

Sometimes it felt as if my back housed a screw, other times, a piece of buckshot. One day I drew a picture of an hourglass. The discomfort was in the narrow place, the gate between all that comes into me and all that goes out.

I talked to the Listener about it. He could hold his hand near my back and feel its crazed energy. He spoke words that helped me understand, then I took the words and ran so much further. I gathered awkward memories and they became congruent, graceful.

It occurred to me that this wasn't a back ailment at all. It was a reflection of the vibration of me.

Dr. Glass classified it as a strain of the trapezius muscle. I got to lie on the table that rolls and jostles the spine, followed by the table where you get hot wet compresses and jolts of electricity. Both were a treat. Then she'd do her reflex analysis and provide the therapy my body seemed to need. In between visits, I did special exercises and took vitamins.

On the days she helped release a "body memory," I was shocked by the things she said to me. No one could guess this stuff, nor was it like the one-size-fits all astrology advice in the newspaper.

"You must be psychic," I said to her. She shook her head no. "I'm just a data collector. It's your body that's speaking."

After nine weeks of therapy she asked me if I thought I was better. "Yes and no. I'm more flexible. I feel discomfort less frequently. But this is my place of tension," I said, reaching around to mid-back. "I still feel something like a bullet."

"What?"

"A bullet."

She studied me for several seconds. "Well, yes. I guess this could be something old," she said, "Something that is coming out because you are ready. You are stronger now."

My fingers itched for that chunk of oak that had popped out of Owen's muscled butt, after a summer of swimming and biking. The hospital had given him an x-ray on the winter day when he'd been impaled. I remember going into the room with him when they placed him on the table under the huge radiation machine.

"Any chance you could be pregnant?" the technician asked.

Owen said nothing. "Any chance you could be pregnant," she asked again. He said nothing.

"Owen," I whispered nervously, "it isn't nice not to answer the lady."

"Mom, I think she's talking to you."

I blushed crimson.

"Any chance you could be pregnant?" she asked.

"Heavens, no."

The x-ray showed no foreign bodies. But the pieces of flooring that emerged a week later, then nine months later, proved the x-ray wrong.

Who knows what we carry in our blood and on our backs that our best diagnostic tools do not reveal?

Who knows when or why symptoms come? Maybe my past had ripened and I was finally ready to greet it, pass it on, or throw it off me.

That day in Dr. Glass's office, face down on the table, the tight midsection of my back finally let go beneath her hands. Snap, crackle, pop. Something came out of my mouth that was both a groan and a sigh.

It was another beginning in a circle of days.

My broker/friend, Alec, told me to call his mother, and he gave me her phone number in Arizona.

"I don't know anyone like her," he said. "She's incredible."

A few weeks later he asked me if I'd talked to her. "No, but I will," I said. He gave me her number again and reminded me that she'd survived more than one go-round with cancer. "But she's never had radiation or chemotherapy," he said.

"Never? Then what does she do?" I asked.

"She prays."

Elaine and I got acquainted over the phone, my through-the-sinus, midwestern accent mingling with her softer one, which carries a trace of something southern. I told her about my encounter with breast cancer, why I was writing, and she agreed to tell me about her healing.

But her story didn't start with a tumor; it started in a bottle, nearly two decades ago.

She had been drinking too much, she said. Alcohol gave her a kind of peace, but it robbed her of strength and substance. Her weight dropped to less than a hundred pounds and she became so weak she couldn't walk—not even from her bed to the bathroom.

"I wanted to die," she recalled. "I saw no brightness in my future."

She was in the hospital, well on her way to realizing that wish. Her organs were shutting down. Her mind already had. She was just awaiting the inevitable.

Then one night she felt a Presence. "I'm convinced it was the Holy Spirit that came to me and said, 'Let's work on this together. If we lean on God, he gives.' That night I placed myself in God's hands."

She did not see herself in the final stages of a disease called alcoholism. She saw herself as weak and worthless, incapable of self-control. She credits this spirit beyond her own intelligence for leading her into an in-treatment program, then Alcoholics Anonymous and a future richer than her dreams.

" 'Let go and let God,' is classic AA. It doesn't sound like much. But there's a lot to it. Live it and you will find less strain and stress in your entire system," she said. "The year I went into AA was the year I started to live."

It wasn't a question of not going to church, not knowing God. She already was an Episcopalian and a well-read woman. It was a matter of developing a faith that could bring her to self-acceptance.

She is seventy now, "kicking higher than I ever have." The God she leaned on didn't just structure her healing. God became her life. God made it possible for her to give up a two-pack-a-day smoking habit and supported her as she encountered cancer more than three times.

Now she rises at 4:00 or 4:30 A.M. for two hours of prayer and meditation. Not because she feels she must, just because it feels right.

"I really like myself now. I know I'm worth something," she said. "But it took me so long to get here. "When I read *Women Who Run with the Wolves* (Clarissa Pinkola Estes' best-seller) I discovered I share this with a lot of women. That book has been a big help. I keep it at my bedside."

Her first encounter with oral cancer was in 1981, about a year after she gave up alcohol. Her husband, a physician, persuaded her to have surgery. But he could not get her to undergo radiation or chemotherapy.

"I saw what radiation did to my mom," Elaine said. "She had throat cancer and died of it."

She also lost all four of her siblings to cancer, as well as other relatives. Doctors could talk to her all day about the benefits of adjuvant therapy. But she wouldn't budge.

"I think it's the treatment that kills people," she said.

Just as difficult as giving up alcohol was giving up tobacco. She knew that squamous cell cancers are fostered by tobacco, but she loved smoking and didn't want to quit. After more cancer appeared in her mouth requiring more surgery, she realized her cigarettes would have to go.

"Yes, it was hard, but God was with me."

She remained cancer-free for a decade. Then in 1990, a tumor sprouted on her neck, seemingly overnight, out of nowhere. Again, she had extensive surgery, lost fifty-two lymph nodes, of which two were positive. But she refused other therapies.

In 1995, her left breast was removed after doctors discovered a number of in situ cancers. Again, she invented her own regimen of follow-up care, recognizing that she had to learn deep relaxation. Each cancer had been preceded by intense family stresses.

"My doctor/husband and doctor/son were furious with me for not taking chemo. My husband said, 'This is like building a house and not putting on a roof.'

" 'But it's not going to rain,' I told him."

In addition to physical therapy, she continued a weekly habit of therapeutic massage, which she swears by. She also takes vitamins and trace minerals daily. But most of her healing work circles around prayer and surrender. Her life in God runs deeper than cancer, which did return, in a different organ, and could again.

A few days after we first talked she sent me some of the prayer cards that she uses, devised by the International Order of St. Luke the Physician:

> Into Your hands I put myself, my soul, my body, my will, my desire—even for healing—my fears my resentments, my ill-feelings, my ambitions. I want, dear Lord, to be what You want me to be—whole in soul and mind and body; that in my whole person I may glorify You, and show forth Your Wholeness. . . . I cannot heal myself; neither can I be healed through anxious prayer.
>
> But when I rest in the silence, healing comes silently and swiftly, so that I find myself whole, before I am aware of any healing taking place.[1]

---

1. Used by permission.

Partners

Dr. James S. Gordon puts up his guard when he hears the term *holistic* linked to other words, including the most common one, *medicine*.

"The word is overused and misused," complained the Washington, DC, physician. *Alternative* is worse. It's a wastebasket term. It sounds like everything one didn't learn in medical school."

It was Saturday, November 22, 1997. I was sitting at the Queen City Club in a seminar titled, "Traditional and Complementary Therapy for Cancer." It was a continuing medical education course for professionals.

I was the guest amateur, invited to speak by my friend, Kathy, an executive in the health-care system that sponsored the event and a champion of holistic approaches.

"Tell them how you see it," she said in one of our phone calls. "We've got a slot on the program."

We both knew this was a rare opportunity. Patients address doctors about as often as kids get to advise school administrators.

Kathy wasn't pushing this for my health, though it was good medicine. She was convinced that the pros needed my words. But she couldn't designate where I'd fit into the program.

I looked at the afternoon's schedule and figured it might be 4:30 P.M. when I got to the podium. First came four medical doctors, two sets of slides, and a break for refreshments.

Dr. Gordon said that instead of *holistic* he advocates the terms *complementary* and *integrative*. But that's semantics. Fact is, he has promoted holistic practices throughout the country and advocated for dramatic changes in health care.

As the founder of the Center for Mind-Body Medicine and a professor at Georgetown University, he searches for responses to disease that incorporate the best of the West, the best of the East, conventional, unconventional.

Yet nearly 80 percent of the clinical work he does "is teaching people approaches they can do themselves"—self-awareness, relaxation, meditation, nutrition.

His investigation of long-term cancer survivors has shown him that their commonality is not a particular medical intervention. Rather, he said, it's found in an attitude of hopefulness, a sense that a health professional and a circle of others are there for them, a spiritual belief system, an exercise regimen and some kind of diet—"it doesn't really matter what."

The standard approach, cultivating "good patients" who will follow strict protocols, hasn't worked very well, he said. Doctors know they aren't getting through to their patients, and this lack of compliance fuels physician burnout.

"If you look at the studies that go into people's medicine cabinets and count pills, the figures are very interesting. Only 18 to 25 percent of people do anything that resembles what their doctor told them to do."

The antidote, Dr. Gordon believes, lies in collaboration with patients. "That's what we're striving for. The new medicine is based on healing partnerships."

It was closer to 5 P.M. and the room was half-empty when I positioned myself behind the microphone with four neatly typed pages. I wanted to talk about the moments when medicine turns magical, when a holy wind blows through examining rooms and operating suites, and doctors and patients are transformed—even if not in ways they anticipated.

But I cleared my throat with none of the exhilaration I had felt while writing. I was wearied by what I'd watched and listened to—the slides and studies, the reluctance to recommend any modality unless researchers from five respected medical centers agree, not to mention the FDA, the NIH, the AMA, the executives of managed care and somebody's uncle in Peoria.

I am aware that medical acceptance can be agonizingly slow in maturing. I understand the need to be blind and double-blind in the search for scientific verity.

But something is missing. It is the same something I had felt after diagnosis, when my surgeon told me that after he did his thing on my breast he would be passing me to an oncologist, radiologist, then plastic surgeons if I opted for reconstruction.

This disease will be vanquished; just fasten your seatbelt.

"Wait," I should have told him. "You need another player. You need me!"

But I didn't know that then. So I said it fifteen months later to the doctors and nurses who were polite enough to tough out that CME course for a few words from a patient:

"Me! Or rather, I need me, since it is my body housing a malignancy, my body that will get cut on, my body that will get dose after dose of caustic chemicals. I need to be consulted, my permission sought and, if possible, my power unleashed. I need to feel that I am taking a tremendous step forward with my life, which, in fact, I am—regardless of the outcome."

Those hangers-on were good listeners. Their silence fueled me.

"Do you suppose that in the same breath that you reveal the presence of cancer you could say 'Welcome'? Could you take my hand, look into my eyes and say that we will be partners? Could you put aside those damn statistics and probabilities and tell me simply that we've got a fighting chance?

"Could you silently affirm the trials and victories of your journey through life, since as a partner I will impact your journey?"

What Dr. Gordon termed *new medicine* is really old medicine. Ancient medicine. Shamans know it. Mothers know it. Those who care lovingly for AIDS patients know it.

Its efficacy may never show up in data, no matter how you slice and dice the human body. But it's already been validated in the yearnings of the heart.

I learned that the day I thought I was going to die of those blood clots. It wasn't my swollen, red arm or the knowledge of a blockade of platelets that got me. It was the piercing pain in my head, the pain that would not be quelled with narcotics.

"Come on in," those good nurses in my oncologist's office said. "We'll work you into the schedule."

They ushered me into an examining room, where I sat five, maybe ten minutes, trying to talk to Hal who had driven me there. But I could no longer resist the pain or the fear. I was crying when the doctor walked in.

"What's going on?" he asked sharply.

I lifted my head like a drunk expecting to see the scowl on a cop's face. I saw concern instead. "I hurt so much," I told him, aware of the novelty of tears. "Could my brain be bleeding?"

"S—," he said, almost under his breath. "Now I'm getting scared."

Then he inhaled and calmly mapped out the rest of the day, explaining how I would go to the hospital, get more tests, get stronger meds, get plasma, and return to his office for removal of the Port-a-cath.

That's what happened. I'm sure it's in my chart.

But search those hundreds of pages and I bet the word s— never appears—at least not as an expletive. Yet it was that unprofessional, thoroughly human remark that ignited hope. He was on my side. Probably always had been.

But I was much too sensitive to his moods, to my memories of a father who was too tired, too busy, too depleted by the practice of medicine. "Tread lightly," my mother would insist after lunch when my father sneaked home for a ten-minute nap to make up for the six hours of sleep he didn't get the night before.

Good children don't ask much of their fathers.

Good patients don't ask much of their doctors. They do what they're told. They swallow their pills. They tread lightly through treatment—unless peculiar ailments get in the way, ailments that scream for attention. Now.

Maybe you will find, as I did, that the person who swears with you and for you creates a healing space, which is intention, then goes with you into the heart of pain, which is holy work, willing to acknowledge a mystery bigger than either of you.

Now you have become partners and you are facing God—only God is hiding, as God always does, in a transparent ribbon of DNA.

Three months after the CME course, I received a call from one of the doctors who had made it to the end of the afternoon. She insisted

I not call her doctor. She had a pressing concern, which had nothing to do with her job.

Her best friend had breast cancer. The surgery had been that morning. She was there, but other friends wouldn't let her see her friend. "Your tears will upset her," they said.

So she went across town, to work. But she couldn't work.

"What should I do?" she asked me. I squeezed the receiver of the phone. She's asking me? What do I know?

I began to babble. But then I recognized that this was a question I still ask myself from time to time: Are tears a burden? Perhaps a drain?

Well, were they? Did I lose something vital when Hal kicked the side of the church, when Betsy's chest heaved as I told her the diagnosis, when Susan cried amid a crowd, when Anne and Megan and Leigh crumbled in the middle of phone calls, when Sian's chin trembled, when Noah insisted, tears hot on his cheeks, that he could not go to school because "somebody needs to stay home and watch you."

No. If those tears took anything from me, it was something that needed to go.

"Don't worry about crying," I told the doctor. "I think she needs to know how much you hurt, how much you care."

"Yes," she said. "That's what I was thinking. I'm on my way."

I went to Mary's house knowing she had a brain tumor.

I went to Claudia's knowing she had diabetes.

I went to Rosie's knowing she had nearly died of toxic shock syndrome.

I thought I knew what their stories would be about. After all, I'd built the frame. I called it "fabulous healing," and since each person had bettered a prognosis or been transformed by loss, all I needed was to slide in the details. Journalism 101.

Yeah, right.

Little prepared me for their private miracles.

"Never go out to an assignment with your story half-written," a crusty, old managing editor said at a staff meeting, not long after I arrived in Cincinnati in 1982. "And never, never write your lead before you do the interview."

I can see him in his pale blue Oxford-cloth shirt, sleeves rolled, collar loosened beneath a tie. Jim was stern, and he was right. A reporter's notion of a good story should never get in the way of the facts.

The facts might be hiding a better one.

Mary

Mary Schoen lives amid purple, violet, lavender, ultramarine and pale yellow, painted on the walls of her three rooms, surrounded by plants growing like crazy, perhaps because she touches and plays with them. In summer, hummingbirds fly up seventeen stories to feast in the jungle on her balcony.

"Everything I do today is what would feel healing," she explained. "Color therapy is very, very powerful."

We were sitting at the dining room table of her Hyde Park apartment, sipping bottled water and getting caught up. I hadn't seen Mary in years or read about her in press releases. In the eighties, she was a peace activist, often shaking a fist at U.S. foreign policy or commuting between Cincinnati and Central America.

"Commuting" sounds too businesslike. It implies a paycheck and benefits. She had none of that, only the support of some local churches and like-minded liberals. She lived on almost nothing. Her job was to document human rights abuses "and walk with the people as they were experiencing trauma."

She found plenty in the battle zones of Nicaragua, Guatemala, and Honduras. Acquaintances kept disappearing. Friends were killed. Children were growing up in the maw of starvation.

A bus exploded in front of her. Soldiers were constantly on the move. During one attack in a tiny village, she lit a candle and watched its flame jump as mortar fire shook her hut. Her prayers were nearly constant.

"How tall are you, Mary?" I asked.

"Five-one," she said. "Why?"

"I'm five-ten. I couldn't have done that. Weren't you scared?" I asked.

She looked at me funny. "Yes, I came to understand terror. But in spite of that I found how to move forward. You know it wouldn't take courage, if you had no fear."

Mary survived Central America's civil wars, wretched plumbing, and ever-present tarantulas. It was here, a hemisphere away in Norwood, Ohio, that she came closest to her own violent end.

"The irony is that I thought I was totally safe here," she said.

She had moved back to Cincinnati in 1990 and taken a job at Xavier University as associate director of the Peace and Justice Program. On a spring night in 1993, a man broke into her apartment and raped her.

It was 3 A.M., and she had been sleeping. At the sight of the attacker, she began reciting the "Our Father" out loud. How she then managed to wriggle free, run out, get a neighbor, come back, and corral the assailant is a mystery she can live with. What she can't live with is the pity the story evokes.

That's why she is reluctant to tell it.

When a friend who learned of the details turned to her and said,

"Oh, Mary, this is going to impact you the rest of your life," Mary put up her hands. "Stop. Yes, it will impact me, but only for the good."

Her challenge has been to trust God and "to trust the process, even if it breaks my body." She decided it was pointless to try to figure out why she was targeted by one man's twisted, drunken lust. "It happened. Now what am I going to do about it?"

She moved to a safer apartment, let the chaos settle, and prepared for trial, which proved almost as devastating as the assault. Even though the rapist was convicted and sentenced to seven years, she felt as if she was being prosecuted for instigating the crime.

"I was a total victim. But then I said, 'No, I refuse to be one.' You don't become a victim by something that happens to you. It's when you decide what you will do with it."

So, Mary, what can you do with it? "You can heal a wound as fast as you can let go of it."

Three years later she came to a similar crossroad. Migraine headaches, distorted vision, an icky sickness. Why?

Doctors found that a tiny, rock-hard tumor was wrapping itself around her pituitary gland and causing her brain to bleed. The tumor was slow-growing and benign, but left unchecked, its damage would be extensive.

She opted against a tricky surgery, though she was willing to take medicine for the rest of her life, alter her lifestyle, and do as much as she could to shrink the tumor and promote healing. But she would not let disease entrap her.

"The rape and the brain tumor have been the most life-changing events for me," she said.

They accelerated her along a spiritual quest she had already begun. She reviewed her childhood, young adulthood, and career choices in a new light. She knew that her social activism in Central America had been prompted by the ongoing abuse of the poor. She passionately admired so many of the people she had met.

But she questioned her effectiveness as an intervenor. "I blamed the system and tried to change the world through impacting externals," she said. "But I got in despair when I came back here. People weren't interested in what was happening in the world. People were dying and they didn't care."

When the rape occurred and again when the tumor was diagnosed, she realized she would not be saved by other victims. She searched her memory for victors. Faces of people she'd met in Central America came flooding back.

In particular, there was a toothless mother, so poor she had only two days' worth of rice and two chickens, yet seven mouths to feed. When Mary and a friend appeared, the woman insisted on killing one of the chickens to give them a special meal. Mary tried hard to talk her out of it.

"But she was smiling as she cooked."

Mary saw this as an example of "trusting the process." She realized "everything can be empowering, if you let it be."

Mary left Xavier in the fall of 1996 to teach Transformational Breath, a breathing technique that facilitated her own healing, and to sell a nutritional supplement called Body Wise. She is thinner, stronger, healthier, happier, she says, than she ever has been. She's giving up her distrust of money and wealthy people and any belief system that identifies with victims and glorifies their wounds.

Claudia

Claudia Bernard lives and works in the upstairs of a remodeled carriage house. It's just one room in Mt. Lookout, smaller than any dwelling she previously occupied; yet she is remarkably content.

In spring, trees enclose her in green, reminding her a little of the two acres she used to own in Anderson Township. But that was a decade and a different lifetime ago.

A friend who has known her for years said to her: "You're more who you are than you ever were."

"I used to not be true to myself," Claudia explained. "I used to be true to my image. Now I don't have an image."

She has come to this point of equilibrium through terrific loss. It began in 1988 when her husband of twenty years left her. They divorced. She lost the house. Her car was totaled. She broke her ankle, was attacked by a dog, then she was diagnosed with insulin-dependent diabetes.

All came tumbling down within two years.

In the beginning of the end, when she was a displaced wife who saw no future for herself, she would lie on the couch and pray: "Please don't let me wake up."

Claudia's candor surprised me. We were sitting at her one and only table, sipping hot lemon water out of porcelain cups. We'd never met before but had talked on the phone, and I'd heard good things about her work as a craniosacral therapist.

The techniques she uses are aimed at evaluating and harmonizing the body's craniosacral system. It is recommended for people with headaches, neck and back pain, eye dysfunctions, dyslexia, chronic middle-ear infections, depression, chronic fatigue, and even some central nervous system disorders.

I assumed she moved into health care after the onset of her diabetes. A number of practitioners I've met describe themselves as "wounded." They know suffering from the inside out.

So does Claudia, but she was already doing craniosacral therapy at Deaconess Hospital when her diabetes was discovered. It was almost a fluke that she had a urine test, the results of which were so astonishing that she and others figured it had to be flawed.

Nine times the normal amount of blood sugar was in her urine—twice as much as the level when hospitalization is required. Most people are unconscious with a mg/dl reading of 900.

"I was actually very functional," she said.

She was tired and tiny, weighing less than 100 pounds, yet eating "like a saint." Organic vegetables, whole grains, and balanced proteins may have saved her. Yet her situation was critical. Her blood sugar was going up. She would have to be hospitalized.

But the five physicians with whom she worked could not convince her. She simply refused. After a heated exchange with one of them, a woman doctor said, "Okay. But you call me at 6:30 every morning and I'll tell you how much insulin to take."

When Claudia retells it, eight years later, she still shakes her head in wonder. "I couldn't believe that someone would do that for me. My heart cracked open and melted.

"My whole life changed. My healing, on the deepest level, was getting to be mothered by her."

Claudia was surprised when she discovered feelings for this woman that she had only known with men. "Linda and I played the relationship out romantically. She provided the sweetness in life that I was missing.

"But Linda had her own troubles. In 1992, she committed suicide."

At the time, Linda was working a job in another state. She'd been tired and depressed, struggling with remnants of a difficult childhood and probably not eating well.

Claudia's new loss made her other ones seem small. She describes it with tears and smiles.

"I'm just glad I had her for a while," she said. "I wouldn't give up a minute with her."

Looking back further than a decade she remembers how much scorn she had for people who took their lives, or those who wanted to. Then she's reminded of the times she lay on her couch hoping to slip away in sleep.

"What I really wanted was a way to commit suicide that no one would know about, and that wouldn't be too traumatic."

Was her prayer answered?

Sort of. She believes that her pancreas, the gland responsible for insulin production, gave her just what she wanted. A way out. A disease, which if unattended to, brings a swift death.

"With insulin and syringes, it's like having a loaded gun around," she said. "My belief is that this condition is serving me in a psychological, emotional way. It makes it safe for me to stay here, because I could go."

Claudia doesn't push the idea. "I don't mean to imply that everybody's conditions are like mine."

She doesn't want to be diabetic. In fact, she dreams and schemes of being "the first person on the planet to get off insulin."

But already she is off judgment and arrogance and attitudes that kept people at a distance. She's become humble, she said, and is so much happier. So are the people around her, she guesses.

"I have a very simple lifestyle. I feel like I'm in alignment with all the parts. I'm not doing anything that feels out of integrity."

Rosie

On the night Rosie Miller came close to death, infection was rioting through her blood.

Pneumonia entered both lungs. Meningitis besieged her brain. Her nervous system jammed and her heart lumbered toward defeat.

"You will have to decide whether I live or die," she said to her best friend, haltingly combining words. "It's no longer my decision."

During the coma that followed, when she was supposed to hear nothing, but heard everything, the lead doctor informed her family and members of her religious community, "She will not last the night."

Sister Rosie, a member of the Sisters of St. Francis of Oldenburg, Indiana, was about to become a casualty of toxic shock syndrome. She was thirty-five.

Instead, she survived and, despite predictions to the contrary, recovered fully. She is now a teacher of theology and yoga and a practitioner of healing touch therapy.

But hers was no tabloid miracle. It unfolded in painfully slow-time. She had to mix the heaven of death with the hell of reentry.

We sat twice together at a tiny table in Rosie's living room with mugs of tea that grew cold. There were so many visceral details that at one point I excused myself, afraid that I was going to faint.

I returned a third time to her big house in Norwood to watch her do healing touch on Mary Schoen, whom she has treated many times for her brain tumor. It was then I began to understand the triumph of life in Rosie, how she can fill an ordinary room with something delicious.

She works mainly in silence, her head tilted, her eyes focused on I don't know what. Her delicate hands brush the air about six inches above Mary; they never make contact. Her voice is barely audible, yet her words are intimate, confident.

Mary interrupts the silence. "Something is draining in my leg. It feels like it's getting longer. I can feel shifts in my head, too."

Rosie nods. When her hands discern an imbalance of energy that she can't quite stabilize, she encourages Mary to bring attention to that area, then continue with it in meditation and prayer.

"Yes, I will," said Mary. "The effects are profound."

"To me, true healing is the integration of mind, body, and spirit. It's not curing," Rosie told me. "I can be cured of cancer and not healed, and I can die of cancer and be healed.

"There was a woman, Jane, who had AIDS, who worked with me and lived with me. She came to speak to one of my classes and said, 'AIDS has been my greatest blessing. I learned about unconditional love through AIDS. That was my path.' She died two months later. But she died a healed woman."

Rosie's own dip into death came on February 26, 1985. At that time, more than one hundred American women had already died of toxic shock syndrome, a disease linked to the use of highly absorbent tampons.

Death, she discovered, agreed with her. "It was such a wonderful state of being. I was so peaceful. It was pure bliss."

As her twilight deepened, relatives and fellow nuns paced around the intensive care unit in Lawrenceburg, Indiana. Members of the parish where she was second in command and residents of the town united in intent.

"What I became so aware of is the power of prayer. It kept me alive. I was drawing every ounce of energy from everyone in the room."

Her compromised body did not succumb. A few days later she opened her eyes and said to no one in particular, "I'm so hungry."

She hurt all over. She had double pneumonia, cerebral meningitis, atrophied muscles, and "drop feet syndrome." She could not walk. Physicians doubted she ever would, and they said her heart damage was most likely permanent.

It wasn't enough that prayer had saved her; she would have to summon new forces to recover—forces they could not help her find.

"It was such a lonely time. For a year to eighteen months I had such a struggle with reentry. Although attached and committed, I'd tell my close friends, 'I don't know who I am.' I didn't have any dreams."

Even now, thirteen years later, she continues to integrate the experience into her life and suspects she always will. "It's the wounded healer who has the ability to heal others. We have to work out our own stories."

Certain things promoted recovery: spending a month with her brother's family and being surrounded by his exuberant children; realizing that she needed hours of direct sunlight; taking off a year to attend personal growth programs and to experience a variety of therapies.

Yoga, breath work, intense meditation, dream analysis, journal writing—all helped her come to terms with her sense that nothing in her life was the same. "I kept asking the question, 'Who am I?' I kept putting it out there. I did not know where I was going."

She was still seeking direction when she accepted a job as parish administrator in a town outside of Louisville. During her two years there, she became a certified yoga instructor and "read tons of books on healing." Only then did she realize she was being pulled to a new career. But what? With whom?

The answer that came at first surprised her religious community. She announced she wanted to work with people with advanced AIDS. "I knew that the moment of death is nothing to be afraid of. I wanted to be the voice of affirmation, to say 'I will be here to be your witness.'"

In 1989, she moved to Cincinnati and began teaching in the theology department at Xavier University and working with AIDS Volunteers of Cincinnati (AVOC). That's how she came to know Jane, a single mother who was living in Over the Rhine and struggling to survive.

Rosie took her into her home, nursed her to her death in 1992, and has remained like a second mother to her sons. "Jane became part of the XU community. She enhanced my teaching. It's what made me authentic with my students. I teach as a healer, not an academician."

Other experiences in Italy, India, and Mexico affirmed her in the role of healer, and training in healing touch therapy and spiritual direction have made her finally feel comfortable with the title.

"I believe love heals, but I'm not the ultimate source of love. My task is to keep myself in the most open capacity for love so that I can be a vehicle to invite other people into the healing journey.

"It's not an instant thing. It's a process."

Another Story

As I was leaving Mary's, she stopped me and said she wanted to give me something. "I'd like to give you a chance to tell me your story of healing. That's really important."

I garbled some thanks and said I'd keep that in mind.

Claudia made the same offer. So did Rosie.

Each had no idea that the others had spoken. Nor that follow-up calls were made to make sure I understood. Talking is good, they said. Listening is good. We must do it for each other.

I was glad they recognized that I am more than a woman with a notebook and a pen. I am not shy about talking. But I didn't know where my story began or ended. I couldn't identify its dramatic core, the place where verbs reach out and grab like those trees in *The Wizard of Oz*.

I couldn't even say whether my healing has happened or is about to happen. All I knew was that I had to get home, settle into a comfortable chair, and listen to my own story.

Redemption

I went in search of Mary Jean this morning. Not for her sake—she's been dead for more than a decade—but for mine.

My first pass through the boxes in my basement yielded nothing except dust on my jeans and the first sneezes of an allergy attack. But I will look again.

I need to measure the me of now, who has experienced breast cancer, against the me of then, a young reporter writing about a woman who would be carried to her death by breast cancer. I knew nothing about it then.

Of course I tried to educate myself in the ways I had been taught. Government statistics. Trend studies. Case management. Doctor interviews. But mostly I talked to her, week after week, for months.

I watched her wear new wigs and bold colors to express courage and hopefulness, then finally the whites and pinks of resignation as she became tethered to an oxygen tank at home.

A few days before her death I went to University Hospital to say good-bye. I was so unsure of myself around her grown kids, almost apologetic for being there. Me: bringing closure to a story. The buzzard circling closer.

Or maybe I misinterpreted their silence. I have always carried guilt while nosing into other people's losses without a stake in their pain. I'm not sure I'll ever get over the voyeurism of news gathering.

No matter that she and her coworkers had sought me out to interview her for a documentary that was shot, but never edited into completed form. No matter that Mary Jean wanted me to write the story she should have written herself.

It was because of her children and grandchildren and other people with cancer that she exposed her hopes for a treatment that didn't work and ultimately her fears of dying. She wanted a rare thing made from her suffering.

But that's not why I went to find the series I wrote. I am not expiating guilt. I want to find my nut graph—the words in a newspaper story that reveal its food. Nut graphs bring on the ah-ha moment, when readers discover why this thing exists and consider whether they want to consume it.

Where did I place the nut? Was it in a sentimental place or an angry one?

I remember that I was putting flesh on a statistic: A real woman dying in her fifties of a much too prevalent disease. But did I play a long, slow victim's lament?

I suspect it. More than half of the stories I have ever written carry that music. I seemed to spread it through my orbit, then, playing like a Pied Piper, I attracted people to me.

The awful power of the victim is the vacuum, the need to suck greater negativity to oneself to justify the perception that one has been wronged.

I can remember the satisfaction in finding a worthy victim of an accident or disease, a good person getting screwed by a bureaucracy. It didn't matter by whom or what.

I would call Paul from the office and tell him I'd be late for dinner. He'd hear the strain and excitement in my voice. "How far along are you?"

"Well, I've only written three paragraphs, but it's coming."

Something in me identified with victims. I could enter into their wounds, shudder about the injustice of their situations. But I wasn't the only one. Wounds are the mashed potatoes of the news business; we stuff our cheeks and still can't get enough.

I won't write those stories again. Not in the same way.

My cancer has shown me we are so much bigger than our wounds. My cancer told me to look elsewhere, to get moving.

On my second trip to the basement I found boxes of old files I should have thrown out long ago. I noticed that if I turned a box in one direction I saw such headings as: Christopher Columbus, solid waste, safe food, Lower Price Hill, Mapplethorpe, covered bridges, and if I turned it the other way: Potter Stewart, nuclear power, anorexia, simple living, Warhol, teenage pregnancy. I have trouble parting with decent file folders, so I have held onto eighty pounds of notes, now frosted with mildew, for two pounds of folders.

My filing method meant I had to open each one, pick through notes, clips, and printouts to determine which heading actually represented its contents. I found stories about people I couldn't remember meeting. I read over names I sort of recognized. Rarely could I conjure a face to go with them. Long stories that I'd spent weeks researching were the eeriest. I saw notebooks filled with my handwriting. I saw my byline on the top of long columns of type. But I felt as if I was reading those stories for the first time, though my vested interest ran deeper.

What happened to the information that once occupied my mind? When Henry David Thoreau went to Walden Pond, he said he wanted to live authentically. When he left, he said he had other lives to live—just as authentically, I suspect.

I know that feeling of detachment. It's as if I have passed through several lifetimes with the illusion of living only one.

Inside a dark folder I found a tiny silver spider, almost transparent, as rare as any orchid at Krohn Conservatory, and still crawling. Inside another I found the text of a 1984 speech delivered by a Brandeis University professor, "Four Steps on the Road to Invalidity—the Denial of Sexuality, Anger, Vulnerability, and Potentiality."

On the cover of his sixteen-page vita, I had scrawled that the author was "a medical sociologist, wheelchair-bound." He gave an address at a local conference of social workers and therapists. I'd probably been sent out to get a "quick and dirty"—newsroom jargon for a short piece, obtained without much digging. I don't know why we call them "dirty," perhaps because it lends an air of intrigue to a story the editor considers merely space-filler.

I leafed through the old speech. The biggest challenge for a person with a chronic or disabling disease, the professor said, is finding "a path between denial and self-pity." Various social pressures make admissions of vulnerability difficult.

In describing prohibitions against crying, he noted that "the fear is that once started, it, like self-pity, will never stop. My own observation is that those people with an oversupply of tears are the ones who have been unable to mourn their losses fully, especially when they first occurred. As a result, they leak and mourn a little bit all the time."

I tossed the speech aside, but found myself talking to it during the afternoon. Me, with a one-page vita, told the professor with a sixteen-page one that people with an undersupply of tears may be just as unable to mourn their losses fully. Some people he knows may be too watery. But I know others who are gunked up, full of salt and mucus.

I remembered leaving Mary Jean's house in Madeira one afternoon, a few days after I'd had another miscarriage. My first would-be child, wondrously similar to a sea horse, I'd flushed down the toilet amid clots of blood and muffled screams. Nothing had prepared me for such vulnerability.

The second would-be child had been sucked out at the hospital—less trauma, less blood, but just as much heartache.

What have I done? Why can't I have children? I sobbed alone in my car, traveling south on Interstate 71.

I had not told Mary Jean about the miscarriage. What was a twelve-week-old fetus compared to a woman's life? In those days I subscribed to a hierarchy of misery, and I decided my dashed hopes didn't rate communion. Besides, I was a reporter, wasn't I? My job was to watch other people, listen to them, record their stories, not allow our lives or losses to mingle. I began to believe this strange configuration, accepting a second-class status. I swept my emotions to the periphery, shrugged off the import of my actions, decided a recorder's life was a full one, even if it didn't quite feel that way.

In my basement, I collected notebooks filled with other people's ideas, their trials, their triumphs. In my breasts, I collected tears.

The same disease that told me to stop looking for people with worthier wounds and saltier tears said the time has come. Open the dam. Let them spill. And then you will want to move on.

In such paradoxes I find my healing.

I like tulips.

She likes tulips.

I like her.

I reach down to pluck it, but it won't snap. Its stalk is stronger than the hands of a four-year-old.

I pull harder, hurriedly, straining with arms and legs.

The earth lets go and it all comes—the pale part that should be underground and the broken bulb.

I know this isn't right, but I want her to have it, flaming orange on the outside, yellow-streaked inside, with that furry black stamen.

My mother is talking with another woman in the church parking lot. They take no notice of me, even when I tug lightly on her skirt. I wait but I can not wait.

"Look, Mommy. Look what I have for you."

She never sees the orange petals, the cup with a zig-zag top that I draw for her on rough manila sheets. She only sees the bulb displaced, a plant stolen from the border that rims the sidewalk. Her face darkens and her words lash, "Camilla, how could you!"

In the face of the other woman, I go dumb. I run to the spot where I'd taken it, scratch in the earth and put it back, head bowed to hide the water in my eyes.

But the earth does not want it.

The tulip falls.

It was then I tasted the briny pain of love—how it hallows, how it hollows.

Unanswered Question

I will ask the question I could not ask: Why was I not with her in her suffering, in her dying, in her passage?

It had something to do with memories. Someone said we would not want to remember her this way, locked in a coma, in constant convulsion, her body tossed like a dead, white fish on stormy seas.

"Preserve the good memories of your mother."

But she is in me. Both bad and good. Tyrant and liberator. I cannot control my remembering. This organ, wherever it is, in the mind or the heart, is autonomic. Diabolic. And divine.

So now I go to that hospital room in Indianapolis. I push past the nurse who found me beating on a wall and tried to steer me into the visitors' lounge. I lower the metal rail on her bed. The weight of my body sinks in beside her.

I do not tell her, as I did then, what I will become, how she will be proud of me. I do not need to see a star of recognition shining in her eyes.

I part the hair on her forehead. I kiss it. I tell her she is the perfect mother, the perfect friend. Perfect, yet imperfect.

I tell her I have made a home. It is my home and she is welcome.

I hold her hands and follow the paths of her veins. And lying close, I whisper so only she can hear: I can take this. I can let you go. Again, if I must.

But only if I can write it. Without words I cannot live.

Unfinished Business

Dear Paul,

I have placed our back taxes, in an orderly fashion, in black filing cases at the bottom of the basement stairs. I didn't buy black on purpose. It was the color du jour at Big Lots. But it is a fitting reminder that the business transactions of our lives, once completed, are dead matter.

I think, for you, they're dead while still alive. It's one of your most maddening, yet admirable traits—a thorough disinterest in finance, official obligations, and monetary gain. You are as free from greed as anyone I know.

If I die before you, the date you must circle is April 15. File the taxes on time.

Do you remember the year we got in a panic because it was March 14 and we thought the deadline was March 15? Babes in the woods, we were.

Are we still? I don't know. Isn't it strange how we can't see our shadows at high noon, and yet it's always at high noon that we are called to account for ourselves?

I am writing this as if my death were close. It is. So is yours. So is everyone's. But we don't conduct ourselves out of that awareness. We don't make our happiness a priority.

We also fail to acknowledge the many deaths and rebirths tucked within the garments of our lives.

That became clear to me when I began to worry about that call from my boss. My rational response, "What could he need?" was upstaged by an irrational one, "What could he do to me?"

The answer is 'nothing,' not because my job is secure (no one's is), but because I feel, in my bones, that I can accept anything. What I dread is the residue of big change. It's a deep sadness, inexplicably more familiar than my own name.

I have been walking the rim of this canyon for days. You know. You've watched. You even sang "Lonesome Valley" with me. But there are certain places I do have to go alone. Certain burdens I must carry or unload.

I am too full of metaphors, but that is the way I see life—always through a screen of sensation, past experience or fable. Dreams provide another screen. They say to me, "Let me show you what this feeling (of hope, challenge, dread, risk, whatever) is about. It's as if. . . ." And the movie rolls.

The "as if" is crucial. It's the lever that lifts what would be a meaningless equation into a meaningful simile.

Grammarians scold us if we mix metaphors or resort to them too often—the offense I confess to committing. But they don't say that a weary cliché is better than none, if it begins to reveal a personal truth.

So bear with me. I feel that my task now is to take off my shoes, stand upon the earth, and sink myself into the strong, balanced, core energy of belonging. I need to be firmly placed, while confronting displacement—the fear of it, the temptation.

Sometimes I don't want to stand, but to disappear. I have no death wish. I really don't. Yet I feel a kinship with the spirit in things that longs for no-thing.

I hear a voice in the marble baptismal font at church. It whispers, "Free me." I sit at a bonfire and watch fire consume a log in orange and purple and blue. The wood sighs and sputters, "Beautiful." I watch geese in flight and wonder, with heart on tiptoe, "Going home?"

It has occurred to me that those mutant cells we call cancer are bit players in this internal drama. I remember when Claudia explained this to me in reference to her diabetes. I was astonished, maybe skeptical. Not so much anymore.

Lynn asked me today, "Is it that we learn to take nothing for granted or everything? Which is it? You've been there, what do you think?"

I have not been there enough. I don't know. One voice says, "Take nothing for granted." This is the path of gratitude. Another voice says, "God provides. Take everything for granted." This is the path of miracles.

But one could also be the path of hesitation; the other of forgetfulness. Is there really an either/or?

I want to live out of gratitude, in that open field. But I know if I did not forget, not take so much for granted, I would not experience disillusionment. Contrary to popular opinion, the loss of illusions is both grievous and ecstatic.

It is one of the ways we suffer ourselves to abiding knowledge.

Please try to explain this to the boys.

Please tell them that each person is a solar system. The challenge of being human is to travel to the farthest ends of your own galaxy, circle the sun, count the moons, know as many planets and stars as you can. Close your eyes and sway with the power of intersecting solar systems. This power is as irresistible as gravity, whether your eyes are open or shut. But then wait—wait until you feel a subtle, unifying hum.

This is the beginning of compassion. Not sympathy, the ache that friends experience, but compassion—discovering that your enemy's pulse sounds so much like yours.

I have done this only once or twice.

Tell Robin that I will still run with her through the fields. I will bike with her to the bridge when the moon is setting, the mist rising, and the sun about to burst through. I will know better the songs of the birds and the names of the wildflowers and I will place the information in her right ear.

Tell Hal to keep pointing to the North Star. So many people can't even find the Big Dipper.

Tell my guardian angel I will guard her.

Tell my many beloved sisters to keep company.

Tell my brothers they are strongest in tenderness, and if they don't believe it, they could study the reproductive system of the red cedar. Hint: For a few days its cone is sticky and yellow and garishly exposed.

I sleep. I dream: I'm in a science lab I don't remembering registering for. We are learning mummification. We work in teams. Another team is further along than mine. My attention is divided. At every step of the way, the teaching assistant demands more money. Somebody tries to rip me off. I am annoyed. I haven't even gotten to do any of the work. Besides it's all sequential, strange and boring.

What folly, the dream seems to say. As if something as personal and precious as preparing for death could be learned in a class!

The images eye me strangely after waking. Where did they come from?

Then I flip them, like that stone we have in the upstairs bathroom, on which somebody painted, "Turn me over." Remember what it says on the other side? "Oh, that feels good."

Now the dream begins to speak to me, kindly, but pointedly: As if something as personal and precious as living could be cut up and distributed! As if one's business could ever be finished!

Who am I to try to pass off my truths as Truth?

I cannot speak for others. I cannot own them, even in my mind, nor can I associate them with me if they do not desire the association.

I can't nail a raindrop to a pine needle.

I can only speak for myself. Own myself. Witness the world in movement around me. It will keep moving, whether I am here or not.

Is that why my heart feels sometimes like a pool of sadness? Is that why I keep writing?

I don't know. But I've found my open road: I pose the questions. I bear witness.

That is enough.